PRAISE FOR

Into a Jewish Holiday Year with Yoga

"Rabbi Tara Feldman and Sharon Epstein have combined their extensive knowledge of Judaism and yoga to present the enormous, multidimensional world of the Jewish holidays with masterful simplicity, beauty, clarity, and depth."

—DIANE BLOOMFIELD, author, *Torah Yoga: Experiencing Jewish Wisdom through Classic Postures*

"Working with one's body is critical to a fruitful, spiritual practice. If you're wondering how, this beautiful, accessible book will take you there."

—RABBI MIKE COMINS, author, *Making Prayer Real: Why Prayer is Difficult and What to Do About It* and *A Wild Faith: Jewish Ways into Wilderness; Wilderness Ways into Judaism*

"This book is a a symphony; an essential guide to any and all of us for whom spiritual life is a fully embodied experience. With the Jewish calendar as our map, Sharon and Tara guide us through multiple entry points—movement, meditation, and journaling—so that we may find the personal relevance that the holiday themes hold for each of us. The suggested postures for each holiday are thoughtfully presented, and the invitation to create our own theme-based yoga practices gives us the chance as practitioners and guides to come back to this book year after year."

—JULIE EMDEN, founding director, Embodied Jewish Learning

"Sharon and Rabbi Tara have created a well-designed approach to help you integrate yoga with Jewish festivals. More people than ever before are looking for a meaningful way to explore the mind-body connection within a Torah context, and this is a helpful tool in that journey. How can we experience Judaism in our body? Now is the time to start!"

—MARCUS J. FREED, author, *The Festive Sutras: A Yogi's Guide to Shabbat & Jewish Festivals*; co-founder of the Jewish Yoga Network

PRAISE FOR
Into a Jewish Holiday Year with Yoga

"This book provides space for introspection, inquiry, and spiritual exploration through the lens of yoga. The text and prompts are accessible for a seeker of any age hoping to dig deeper into their practice."

—Amanda Greenawalt, advancement director, B'nai Jeshurun, NYC

"*Into a Jewish Holiday Year with Yoga* is a beautiful and accessible guide to moving through the Jewish year cycle with essentials of both Jewish spiritual practice and yoga. Tara and Sharon offer foundational insights and inspiration for embodied spiritual practice that draw upon their combined years of practice and teaching. This book is a powerfully integrated approach to moving through the Jewish year cycle!"

—Rabbi Myriam Klotz, RYT, founding co-director of
Yoga and Jewish Spirituality Teacher Training,
Institute for Jewish Spirituality, NYC & Philadelphia, PA

"If our holidays are truly to land in us, we have to prepare to enter them, defenses down. But how? This honest, integrated, and thoughtful book is just such a prescription for finding the calendar in us and finding ourselves in the calendar. A gift."

—Noa Kushner, founding rabbi, The Kitchen, San Francisco, CA

"Exquisite and breathtaking. Beautifully crafted, rich in content and easy to access. Finally—a holistic approach aligning mind, body and soul."

—Laurie Phillips, Founder and Director, Beineinu, Between Us, NYC

"Tara and Sharon's rich, warm analysis serves as a reminder of the countless ways that Jewish and yogic traditions can beautify and enhance each other. Using their book will inspire rabbinical students and yoga teachers to both enrich their communal offerings and deepen their personal spiritual practice."

—Rebecca Thau, HUC-JIR rabbinical student and yoga teacher

Into a Jewish Holiday Year with Yoga

A Workbook and Guided Journey for Body, Mind, and Soul

Rabbi Tara Feldman and Sharon Epstein

Illustrations by Adam J. Schiff

Into a Jewish Holiday Year with Yoga
©2021 Rabbi Tara Feldman and Sharon Epstein

The content of this book is for educational purposes only. Each person's physical, emotional, and spiritual condition is unique. Before using this book, you may wish to consult with your healthcare provider. By using this book, you acknowledge and agree that when practicing yoga physical injury is possible. You assume the risk and responsibility for any such results.

Book design and production by Schultz Yakovetz Judaica (www.schultzyakovetz.com).

Image credits:
Author photo by Barbara Herman.
Yoga illustrations by Adam J. Schiff.
Front cover illustration: CrushPixel #711089 by picoStudio.
Holiday illustrations: pp. 2, 18, 26, 34, 42, 58, 74: CreativeFabrica #8574344 (adapted) by BSD Studio; p. 6: Adobe Stock #346240696 by BSD Studio; p. 10: Adobe Stock #140482326 by BSD Studio; p. 50: Adobe Stock #224174754 by BSD Studio; p. 66: Adobe Stock #241823914 by Olga; p. 82: Adobe Stock #401250183 (adapted) by BSD Studio; p. 90: Adobe Stock #228037318 (adapted) by Vector Tradition.

ISBN 979-8-9850271-0-5

Printed in the United States of America.
Published by Lev Shalem Yoga, Great Neck, NY (www.LevShalemYoga.com).

This book is dedicated to my parents, Lillian and Morton Alpert, for their abundant love and support. Their insistence that I attend Hebrew school and become a Bat Mitzvah, at a time when few girls were encouraged to do so, empowered me to strengthen my Jewish identity. Simultaneously, my parents gave me the opportunity to delight and to delve into the study of dance. These experiences have made a lasting imprint on my body, mind, and soul, for which I will be forever grateful.

This book is a tribute to the many dance and yoga teachers who have inspired me in the past and continue to nurture me on my journey. Also, it is an offering for those who seek enrichment through integrating the treasures of Jewish life with the healing and transformative wisdom of yoga.

—Sharon Epstein

This book is dedicated to my "Grandma Kate," Kathryn Mullowny, who danced for choreographer George Balanchine and, through her life as a ballet teacher, set a shining example of embodied spirituality. This book is dedicated, as well, to my parents, Judith Himber and Victor Himber *z"l*, and Susan Sherwin and Richmond Campbell, for sparking my love of movement and igniting my quest for intellectual and spiritual fulfillment. They have nourished that flame through their unwavering support and through the example of their own lives.

Finally, this book is dedicated to my life partner, Rabbi Meir Feldman, for sharing the journey and for giving me encouragement and space to explore my own path of spiritual expression. Meir's passion for Torah, Hebrew, prayer, and Israel infuses my life with vitality. His devotion to family is my foundation. Meir's ability to live courageously is my inspiration.

—Tara Feldman

Contents

Foreword

More than thirty years ago, after five years of immersion in Torah study in Jerusalem, I had a dream where I saw three African women in traditional dress dancing. I knew that their dance was prayer. I woke up realizing that I needed to pray and learn Torah, not only with my words and mind, but with my whole body.

When I was a young girl I would watch my sister doing yoga. I was drawn to the spiritual beauty of the postures. I felt then that one day I would do yoga. After my dancing-prayer-dream, I began to practice yoga. With yoga, I discovered and experienced the Torah wisdom that had been in my mind, now dancing within my body. Torah Yoga was born.

Since that time, I have continued to occupy myself daily in the deep study of Torah and the practice of yoga. I have developed, taught and written about Torah Yoga. My book, *Torah Yoga: Experiencing Jewish Wisdom Though Classic Postures*, was published in 2004.

With Torah Yoga, through the study of Jewish wisdom together with the practice of yoga, yoga postures become gateways to expanding Torah consciousness. Torah teachings illuminate hidden inner worlds. One of my greatest yoga teachers, Faeq Biria, told me that the truest yoga is yoga that leads one to a deeper connection to oneself. "If you are Jewish," he said, "yoga will deepen your connection to your Jewish soul."

When I began exploring Torah Yoga, I didn't know anyone who was connecting Torah and yoga. I discovered, however, that the connection of Torah to the body is not a new one. Our wise Rabbis of the Zohar and Midrash teach that Torah existed even before creation. It was God's blueprint for all reality. Therefore everything in creation, including our bodies, has Torah encoded in it.

The Chassidic Rabbi Sfat Emet teaches; "The words of Torah are engraved in the body of a person, but they are hidden and need to be discovered. Of course they are!" he exclaims, "because with Torah, God created the world."

The seeds of Torah Yoga, planted in creation, began to blossom with Abraham, the first father of the Jewish people. We find hints to Torah Yoga in the letters of Abraham's Hebrew name אברהם (Avraham). In Torah, names are enormously significant. A person's name contains the essence of his soul and his purpose in life. Rabbi Moshe Cordovero teaches that the deepest spiritual secrets are found in the Hebrew letters. Every Hebrew letter has a number connected to it. The number equivalent of the letters in Abraham's name is 248. Our sages teach that there are 248 limbs in the human body. There are also 248 positive מצוות (*mitzvot*) in the Torah. As well as meaning "commandment," *mitzvah* also means "connector." Each commandment is designed to connect the actions of our 248 limbs with holiness. This numerical connection between Abraham, the body, and mitzvot, hints to the essential purpose of the Jewish people; to connect the physical to the spiritual; to discover God, not only in our souls, but in our bodies, and through our actions.

If connecting Torah to the body is as old as creation, why is Torah Yoga a new and often surprising idea? According to Rabbi Abraham Isaac HaCohen Kook, it is because of exile. When the Jewish people were exiled from the land of Israel, they became disconnected from their bodies. Rav Kook teaches that when the Jews return to their land as a people, they will return to their bodies as individuals. In the land of Israel, the connection between the spiritual and physical can fully flower.

That is why, although Torah Yoga has its roots in the oldest of ideas, it was hidden for many years. Now that the Jewish people have begun to return to their land, we are re-awakening the ancient body-soul connection. At the time that I began to see glimpses of Torah Yoga, many others were having similar visions. I began to offer classes to students who were delighted to include their body in their Torah study, and to practice yoga that inspired their Jewish soul. Torah Yoga also draws students from other faiths who connect to the treasure chest of Jewish wisdom.

In 2018, I received an email from Sharon Epstein telling me that she was inspired by my book *Torah Yoga* and was using it as a resource at the Jewish Yoga school that she and her rabbi, Tara Feldman, had set up in Great Neck, New York. Sharon asked if I would like to meet Rabbi Tara, who was coming on a six-month sabbatical to Israel with her family. We met at a coffee shop in Jerusalem and spoke for hours about our shared passion for Jewish wisdom and its essential connection to the body. When Tara spoke, I felt I was hearing the words of my own soul articulated. Tara and I also passionately share the vision of deepening this body/soul work in Israel. Tara and her family are now moving to Israel, and will live across the street from my home. In 2020 I was pleased to teach in Tara and Sharon's Jewish Yoga school.

Rabbi Tara and Sharon's gorgeous new book adds greatly to the growing Torah Yoga garden. These seasoned teachers have combined their extensive knowledge of Judaism and yoga to present the enormous, multidimensional world of the Jewish holidays with masterful simplicity, beauty, clarity, and depth.

Each chapter begins by rooting us in the traditions of the holiday. Essential Hebrew words are artistically presented בעברית (*b'ivrit*), in Hebrew, so all can enjoy the beauty of the Hebrew language and meditate on its secrets. Through well-instructed yoga postures, playful illustrations, and guided meditations, this book is a wonderful guide to the life-enhancing wisdom planted within us at the time of creation.

— Diane Bloomfield
October 2021

Diane Bloomfeld is the author of Torah Yoga: Experiencing Jewish Wisdom through Classic Postures *(2004). She is the creator of Torah Yoga and teaches it throughout North America, Israel, and Western Europe.*

Acknowledgments

A heartfelt thank you to everyone who gave their time, talent, expertise, and support with this book project.

Thank you to Jenn Still-Schiff and Len Schiff for their encouragement and creative input, and to our talented young illustrator, Adam J. Schiff. We offer much gratitude, as well, to our patient, generous, and skilled book designer, Erica Schultz Yakovetz, and to our copy editor Sheri ArbitalJacoby.

Thank you to Ewa Abrams, Michael Freeman, Linda Friedner, Laurie Haber, Nina Koppelman, Barbara Herman, Arthur Kurzweil, and Genia Taub for their abundant kindness and knowledge in response to all of our questions, requests, ideas and concerns. Our gratitude to Elanit Rabbani-Rodriguez for inspiring and sharing the name *Lev Shalem Yoga*. Thanks to Penina Mazor and Shy Kedmi for help with Hebrew language questions.

Thank you to all the students, trainees, and teachers who consistently participated and were involved with Jewish Yoga School programs over the years. Thank you to the Sisterhood and congregants at Temple Beth-El of Great Neck who enthusiastically showed up to our classes and events.

To the Temple Beth-El staff: Dafna Weintraub, Joy Palevsky, Cari Horn, Jonathan Muniz, Nancy Reyes, Sheri ArbitalJacoby, Amanda Greenawalt, Jaqui Wadsworth, Rabbi Devorah Marcus, Cantor Vladimir Lapin, Cantor Adam Davis, and Stu Botwinick who supported, nourished, and cheered our efforts.

Thank you to Rabbi Shefa Gold who granted us permission to enjoy and share her beautiful chants. Thanks to Marie Mularcyzk who brought Shefa's chants to life during our in-person classes with her soulful voice and singing bowl.

Thank you to Diane Bloomfield for being an inspiring friend, author, scholar, and leader in the Jewish yoga world. Thanks to Myriam Klotz and Sheila Peltz Weinberg of The Institute for Jewish Spirituality for the soul-nourishing and transformative retreats and resources. And thank you to Rabbi Mike Comins for the Sinai wilderness retreat which inspired Tara at the start of her Jewish journey.

And finally, a huge thank you to our families: Rabbi Meir, Gavi, and Adina Feldman; and Ron, Matthew, and David Epstein for their patience, encouragement and belief in our project, for their enduring love and for the joy, purpose and meaning they bring into our lives.

Introduction

Sharon recalls an early experience that sparked inner awareness and connection. While joining an Israeli folk dance in her Hebrew school courtyard in Bellerose, New York, energy and movement became an expression of prayer for her. From that time forward, Sharon sensed a spiritual yearning for God, which she pursued through community, dance and the healing arts. Years later, Sharon became a dance therapist and then, drawn to the depth and vitality of yoga, she became a yoga teacher. Sharon was intrigued by teachings from the Hindu, Taoist, and Buddhist traditions. However, as she began to understand yoga more deeply, she felt a gnawing conflict between this spiritual path and Judaism. Sharon wanted to draw upon the profound spiritual wisdom from Eastern philosophy and also revive, not ignore or abandon, her identity as a Jew.

Tara recalls a Sukkot camping trip in the Sinai desert during rabbinical school, which integrated rigorous hiking with in-depth study and contemplation of Jewish text. During this trip, the group ascended one of the rocky desert heights, from which they spotted Mount Sinai. The experience was rooted in the physical while stretching toward transcendence. Inspired by that trip, Tara has continued to seek out and create experiences of embodied spirituality. She believes that building a bridge may provide inspiration to those who have leaned away from Jewish life, assuming that physical-spiritual integration can be experienced only in the yoga studio, at the ashram, on the hiking trail, or at the gym. For Tara, Jewish yoga is a path to unite her joy in movement with her passion for Jewish tradition.

In 2009 when Sharon met Tara, her rabbi at Temple Beth-El of Great Neck, she was excited to rekindle her Jewish studies and collaborate, creating yoga classes inspired by Jewish themes. With Tara as her rabbi and friend, Sharon continues to nourish her spirit, exploring questions and finding resonance between an embodied spiritual practice and her Jewish roots. Through her work with Sharon, Tara finds Jewish yoga to be a resource that opens new dimensions in ancient Jewish teachings, making them accessible to the modern seeker as sources of spiritual sustenance. This book grew out of Sharon and Tara's collaboration, teaching Jewish-themed yoga classes, and leading events, retreats, and teacher training.

Who Will Find Meaning In This Book

Into a Jewish Holiday Year with Yoga is a gateway and guide. The purpose of this book is to add richness, depth, and meaning to the experience of a Jewish holiday year through the practice of yoga. It is adaptable for use in yoga or Judaic settings, for group experiences, or for solitary practice.

Into a Jewish Holiday Year with Yoga is a resource for:

- Yoga practitioners and instructors exploring the integration of yoga with Jewish tradition;
- Educators and community leaders facilitating Jewish experiences in synagogues, schools, community centers, retreats, and summer camps;
- All who seek an expanded, enlivened, and embodied experience of the Jewish holiday year; and
- All who love Judaism and yoga.

The texts, sequences, and ideas found within these pages are designed to be accessible to those who may be new to yoga or Jewish tradition while, at the same time, offering fresh perspectives for experienced yogis and those immersed in Jewish life and learning. Through poses and posture, breath work, guided meditation, Hebrew mantras, and Jewish texts, *Into a Jewish Holiday Year with Yoga* is intended to invigorate the experience of Jewish life—body, mind, and soul.

Where, When, And How to Find Meaning In This Book

While it can be read in a single sitting, *Into a Jewish Holiday Year with Yoga* is designed to be explored over time. Travel with it through the seasons. One's experience of the holidays—their flavors, moods, and wisdom—will change and evolve by revisiting these chapters each year.

Open this book on the yoga mat or in the classroom. Keep it on a bedside table. Use it as a personal visioning and brainstorming tool.

Take each chapter as a whole, incorporating all of its elements, or simply focus on one pose, one meditation, or one text that brings the holiday alive. Mix and match. Treat these pages as a workbook, selecting the aspects that are personally meaningful.

Within Each Chapter

Each chapter includes the following sections:

- **Holiday Traditions,** מָסוֹרֶת הֶחָג, *Masoret HeChag*, an explanation of the basic aspects of the holiday

- **Intentions for the Soul,** כַּוָּנוֹת הַנֶּפֶשׁ, *Kavanot HaNefesh*, a description of the holiday's core spiritual themes

- **Intentions for the Body,** כַּוָּנוֹת הַגּוּף, *Kavanot HaGuf*, a description of how core spiritual themes are expressed by the body through yoga

- **Essential Poses,** תְּנוּעוֹת חִיּוּנִיּוֹת, *T'nu'ot Chiyuniyot*, illustrations and descriptions of suggested central poses for the holiday's yoga practice

- **Your Yoga Sequence,** רֶצֶף תְּנוּעָה, *Retsef T'nu'ah*, a space for taking notes and for expanding upon suggested Essential Poses in order to create a yoga sequence of your own

- **Guided Meditation,** מֶדִיטַצִּיָה מוּדְרֶכֶת, *Meditatziyah Mudrechet*, a meditation and visualization to be offered aloud as others listen—or to be adapted in order to provide a framework for private reflection

- **Journaling,** יוֹמָן, *Yoman*, a space to explore the personal meaning of each holiday in response to guiding questions

Each chapter also includes:

- **A Hebrew Word,** a mantra for guided meditation to be used as a spiritual focal point for the practice of yoga and for reflecting upon the holiday as whole

- **Quotations,** texts from Jewish tradition, to provide grounding and inspiration, at the open and close of each chapter

SACRED LANGUAGE

Hebrew

The depth and power of Jewish tradition is inextricably bound to the beauty and vibrancy of the Hebrew language. Thus, *Into a Jewish Holiday Year with Yoga* draws upon and utilizes an abundance of Hebrew words and phrases, prayers, and source texts. Each chapter also offers a Hebrew word or phrase which expresses an essential aspect of the holiday. Hebrew words are made accessible through translation and transliteration. Both for those familiar with Hebrew and for those new to the language, incorporating Hebrew enriches one's connection to Jewish tradition. Gaze at a Hebrew word, witnessing its shape and beauty. Speak or whisper the word aloud. Notice what arises. Imagine each Hebrew word and letter as a universe unto itself, as a gateway to deeper understanding.

Sanskrit

Sanskrit is the mother tongue of the yoga tradition. This ancient language has an energetic resonance that both deepens and elevates the experience and practice of yoga. The word "yoga" comes from the Sanskrit root *yuj*, meaning "to yoke" or "to join." At its most basic level, this yoking or joining refers to the yogic philosophy of recognizing and uniting opposites into a unified whole. For the purpose of this book, the yoga poses mentioned have been translated from the original Sanskrit into English. A focus on the profound breadth and meaning of Sanskrit is not the expertise of the authors nor the intention or purpose of this book.

Naming the Divine

Jewish tradition utilizes many names for God, both ancient and modern. God's holiest name, indicated by the letters *yud-hey-vav-hey*, is—in fact—unpronounceable. For the purpose of prayer and the reading of scripture, this holiest name is referred to as *Adonai* (My Lord). In everyday speech, the Hebrew word *HaShem*, "the name," allows the speaker to refer to God while maintaining respect for God's sanctity and mystery. Modern day and traditional expressions of God's name include Holy One of Blessing, Source of All Being, *Chavayah* (God of Presence), *Ribono Shel Olam* (Master of the Universe), *Ya* (referring to the *yud* of God's holiest name), and many more variations in both English and Hebrew. No word or phrase can fully capture the essence of the Divine. Therefore, in addressing God, be humble, curious, and creative. Incorporate translations for God's name that balance and reflect both personal inclinations as well as one's wider circle of communal practice.

SACRED TIME

The Jewish Calendar

Jewish time, its holiday cycles and seasons, is defined by a calendar that is both lunar and solar. Each of the 12 Hebrew months lasts 29 or 30 days. In ancient times, Rosh Chodesh (the "head of the month") was announced only after the first sliver of a waxing crescent moon had been sighted in the night sky. Each month and day of the Jewish year begins at sundown. For example, Shabbat which falls on Saturday, begins on Friday evening. Because lunar months are slightly shorter than those in the Gregorian calendar, the Jewish calendar must be adjusted in order to ensure that the holidays remain in sync with nature's annual solar cycles. Thus, about once every three years, Adar II—a second Hebrew month of Adar—is added (similar to the way February 29 is added during leap year on the secular calendar), bringing the total number of months to 13.

A List of Hebrew Months:	Holiday Dates:	
Tishrei	Rosh Hashanah	1st–2nd of Tishrei
	Yom Kippur	10th of Tishrei
	Sukkot	15th–22nd of Tishrei
	Simchat Torah	23rd of Tishrei
Heshvan		
Kislev	Hanukkah	25th of Kislev–3rd of Tevet
Tevet		
Shevat	Tu B'Shevat	15th of Shevat
Adar (Adar II)	Purim	14th of Adar
Nisan	Passover (Pesach)	15th–22nd of Nisan
Iyar	Counting of the Omer	16th of Nisan–5th of Sivan
Sivan	Shavuot	6th–7th of Sivan
Tammuz		
Av	Tisha B'Av	9th of Av
Elul	Elul	1st–29th of Elul

When referring to the secular or Gregorian calendar, Jews use the terms BCE (Before the Common Era) or CE (the Common Era) rather than BC or AD. This book, *Into a Jewish Holiday Year with Yoga*, is being completed in 2021 CE. The year corresponds to 5782 on the Hebrew calendar, indicating in the Jewish imagination the number of years since the creation of the world.

SACRED FOUNDATIONS

Bridging Traditions

Yoga and Judaism represent distinct spiritual paths, each with unique customs, practices, teachings, and beliefs. The goal of this book is not to give the impression that yoga and Judaism are one and the same, nor is it to create contrived parallels between the two. Rather, the aspiration is to use yogic practices to enrich and embody the experience of Jewish tradition.

Judaism does contain elements of physicality, including: the choreography of prayer (standing, bowing, swaying), ritual acts (building a sukkah, cleaning for Passover, carrying a Torah), the physicality of singing, and that of eating and fasting, aspects of Kabbalistic meditation practice, and even Israeli folk dance. Still, for many, especially those in the mainstream, Jewish tradition remains largely inert—cerebral and disengaged from the body, from breath and heart. Thus, *Into a Jewish Holiday Year with Yoga* draws upon yoga to create a holistic, joyful, multifaceted, embodied practice which aspires to bring the Jewish calendar more fully to life.

Yoga's Roots and Definition

Originating in India thousands of years ago, Yoga is the practice of physical postures, breathing exercises, and meditation to promote holistic health in body, mind, and spirit. Yoga encompasses a vast, complex body of knowledge and practice based on physical, metaphysical, and philosophical teachings. Many lineages and styles have evolved over time, especially throughout the 20th century when charismatic and influential gurus and teachers traveled to share their insights, which would eventually reach millions of people worldwide. In the evolution of yogic concepts, various adaptations and interpretations continue to transform yoga, making it popular and accessible to modern practitioners.

The Body as a Sacred Vessel

A new yoga student might arrive at the mat with the intention of becoming more balanced, flexible, and physically able. This utilization of yoga is essential, as it creates the foundation of a healthy and vibrant body. However, this is only the beginning. A deepening yoga practice integrates the realm of the physical with the spiritual, expanding to engage the heart, mind, and soul. The body is a vessel for holy energy. Ultimately, a yogic path reveals layers of conscious connection. Regardless of one's religious context, at its highest frequency yoga offers a gateway toward enlightenment, providing the ability to rise up and help understand and integrate the human experience.

Honoring the Body

Avoid injury by paying respectful attention to the body, mind, and breath. If a history of injury, illness, or other challenges exist, modify, change, or skip poses that are not comfortable or accessible. Aim for the practice to feel pleasant and invigorating, strengthening without strain. Yoga is not competitive. Maintain a relaxed focus. Use good judgment, avoiding anything that feels painful or precarious.

PRACTICES

Essential Yoga Poses and Appendix

In modern day yoga, more than a thousand postures with variations and modifications are available to suit a practitioner's interest and ability. The Essential Poses section found in each chapter offers a curated selection of basic poses which bring out the holiday's themes and essence. These poses are a suggestion and a starting point. The Essential Poses can be used as a short practice unto itself or as a segment within a broader yoga sequence.

Turn to the "Yoga Appendix" at the back of this book (page 97), or find other resources for creating a more extended, personalized Jewish yoga practice.

Illustrations

The yoga illustrations in this book are intentionally human and whimsical. Rather than presenting photographs of practitioners that emphasize exact "perfect" alignment, these chapters aspire to bring out the essence of each pose and express the accessibility of yoga for all.

Breath

A well-rounded yoga practice not only includes postures but also integrates breathing, chanting, meditation, and relaxation. Various yogic breathing techniques may be incorporated before, during, and after a yoga practice. Intentional and full breathing is the practice suggested in the Essential Poses and Guided Meditation sections of this book. For additional information, seek out resources on *pranayama* breathing practices.

Chant

The repetition of sacred words offered through melody opens new portals of consciousness. Chants engage the physical, drawing awareness to the breath and creating a vibration in the body. Chanting with others can deepen communal connection. Offering Hebrew words in chant or song heightens awareness of the infinite meanings contained in the words of Jewish tradition. Chanting allows ancient texts to nourish the soul.

For more information on how to use the chants suggested in this book, see the Resources section that follows.

Meditation

Creating a space for silence and inner reflection will deepen the experience of each holiday's meaning. For this portion of the practice, find a position that is dignified but comfortable. Sit in a chair or on a mat, with or without props. Breathe. Seek the balance of becoming still, yet alert. The Guided Meditation section provides direction on how to drop down into the body for a few moments or an extended period. Draw upon and adapt these offerings to lead others in meditation. Practicing alone? Record and read the suggested prompts and then, with eyes closed, listen to them. Allow silence and sensation to be a pathway for new awareness and insight. New to meditation? Practice self-compassion. If attention and presence should drift, continue to return to the breath and to the mantra: Notice. Breathe. Become present.

RESOURCES

Chants

The "Holiday Chants, Prayers, Songs, and Texts" section at the end of this book suggests a chant, created by Rabbi Shefa Gold, for each holiday. As described in the Practices section above, Hebrew chants powerfully enrich one's practice. Recordings of these chants can be found on Rabbi Gold's website, www.rabbishefagold.com, under Chants and Practices. Footnotes for each chant in the book include a chant-specific link and the English name by which it is identified. To find chants that resonate with you, explore Rabbi Gold's website as well as other resources.

Prayers, Songs, and Sacred Texts

The "Holiday Chants, Prayers, Songs, and Texts" section also includes prayers, source texts, and songs to expand one's holiday observance and yoga practice. These are just a starting point. Use them to enrich your holiday repertoire. Consider them a gateway, an opening to deeper Jewish knowledge and engagement both on and off the mat.

ENRICHMENT

Accompanying Music

Melodies, both traditional and modern, awaken our senses and create a heart-opening atmosphere in which to explore the essence of each holiday. Create a playlist. Consider enlivening the holiday yoga experience with live musicians. Remember, as well, that there are times when silence and the awareness of breath is the best accompaniment.

Props and Setting the Space

Very little equipment is needed for yoga. What is recommended: a clean, warm space, large enough to recline and stretch, and a non-skid surface, such as a yoga mat. Wear comfortable clothing that allows for freedom of movement. Use props such as chairs, walls, blocks, straps, blankets, and cushions for additional support and comfort. Props can be purchased online, but one can be creative and use items found around the house: A belt or tie can substitute as a strap; books can be used in place of blocks. For indoor group classes, an open, well-ventilated space with minimal distractions is optimal. During home practice, choose a room that feels safe and sacred. Consider bringing yoga outdoors, improvising and attuning one's practice to nature's surroundings.

Into a Jewish Holiday Year with Yoga

1
Rosh HaShanah

The Head of the Year

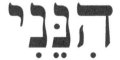

הִנֵּנִי

Hineini • Here I am

Then an angel of God called to him
from heaven: "Abraham! Abraham!"
And he answered, "Hineini. Here I am."

GENESIS 22:11

HOLIDAY TRADITIONS

Beginning Again

- Rosh HaShanah, the Jewish New Year, falls on the first day of the month of Tishrei. This two-day holiday begins a ten-day period called the *Yamim Nora'im,* the Days of Awe or High Holy Days.

- On Rosh HaShanah. Jews gather at synagogue, where the *shofar,* a ram's horn, is sounded 100 times, invoking the themes of *Malchuyot* (God's sovereignty) *Zichronot* (God's remembrance), and *Shofarot* (our hopes for future redemption).

- Torah readings for Rosh HaShanah describe the miraculous announcement of Isaac's birth and his near sacrifice.

- During Rosh HaShanah, Jews engage in the ritual of *tashlich,* casting pieces of bread upon "living water" (a pond, lake, stream, river or ocean) in a gesture of naming and releasing one's sins.

- On Rosh HaShanah, a round *challah* (bread) is eaten, symbolic of the circle of the seasons, and apples are dipped in honey as an expression of hope for sweetness in the year to come.

כַּוָּנוֹת הַנֶּפֶשׁ *Kavanot HaNefesh*

INTENTIONS FOR THE SOUL

Entering the New Year as Our Best Selves

Rosh HaShanah is considered *Yom Harat HaOlam*, the Birthday of the World. It is also known as *Yom HaDin*, the Day of Judgment. Beginning on Rosh HaShanah and continuing through to the end of Yom Kippur, God is said to open the Book of Life in which we pray to be inscribed and sealed. The prayers of Rosh HaShanah invite us into a threefold process of spiritual cleansing and renewal. Through the threefold process of 1. *teshuvah*—repentance (returning to our better selves), 2. *tefillah*—prayer (inner self-examination and communion with God), and 3. *tzedakah*—charity (giving monetary resources to promote the values of *tzedek*—justice, and *hesed*—compassion), we create pathways for renewal and return. The blowing of the shofar signals a spiritual awakening which calls us to embrace the deeper meaning and purpose of our lives and to enter the New Year as our best selves.

The blowing of the shofar signals a spiritual awakening.

כַּוָּנוֹת הַגּוּף *Kavanot HaGuf*

INTENTIONS FOR THE BODY

Showing Up with Vibrant Presence and Energy

In our Rosh HaShanah yoga practice, we prepare ourselves to become present. We recommit to ourselves, our families, our communities, and to God, declaring, "Here I am. *Hineini!*" This yoga practice invites us into the embodied and spiritual experience of "showing up". Our essential postures are the steady, strong, and exuberant **Mountain** and **Extended Mountain Pose**. We stand grounded and upright within ourselves. Let's focus on developing a vibrant presence and energy, ready to be counted, inscribed and sealed for a sweet New Year of blessings, meaning, and purpose.

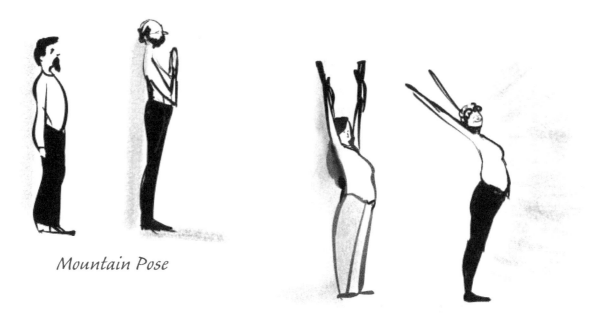

Mountain Pose

Extended Mountain Pose

Mountain Pose

- Become present, standing with both feet planted into the ground. Lengthen the tailbone down toward the heels of the feet and into the earth. Lift the crown of the head upward toward the sky.

- Energetically, feel the alignment of the spine.

- Breathe in fully through the nose and breathe out through the nose several times. Release the arms and sense the shoulder blades on the back, drawing them together. Notice and expand the collar bones. Become alert and erect in **Mountain Pose**. Join the palms of the hands together near the center of the heart.

Extended Mountain Pose

- With an inhale, reach the arms and hands toward the heavens. Relax the shoulders downward while toning the front ribs in toward the spine. Experience the majesty of **Extended Mountain Pose** for 3-5 cycles of deep breath.

- Breathe in and out through the nose. Stand present and willing to faithfully receive whatever blessings and challenges this new year may bring.

- Release the arms and come to a steady, relaxed stance. Smile and acknowledge the light and life within. Whisper, *"Hineni"* (Here I am).

YOUR YOGA SEQUENCE

הִנֵּנִי *Hineini.* Here I am.

Focusing on the Hebrew word above, create and expand upon your own yoga practice. Embody the themes of the holiday.

- a space for divine inspiration & practical ideas -

Find a seat for meditation.
Close the eyes.
With an alert spine, settle into stillness.
Observe the breath.
Notice any sounds. Feel the air on the skin.
Become present.

Breathe in through the nose and out through the mouth. Each outbreath is a means to release tension held in the face, shoulders, or seat. With subtle focus, adjust the body's position in order to be comfortable and to become fully present. Continue to breathe with intention. After each exhalation, whisper the Hebrew word: הִנֵּנִי, "Hineini." Allow for a brief pause before inhaling again.

Now, begin a threefold meditation journey from the past, to the future, to the present.

In the ritual of *tashlich*, we cast bread upon the water as a gesture of releasing sin. Consider this question: As I turn to face the new year, what habit, memory, or current reality do I wish to release, to let go? With each exhalation, let go of the past.

Now envision a goal or dream for the year ahead. Imagine achieving this aspiration. Allow a smile to come to the lips. With each inhalation, invite openness and curiosity. With each exhalation, see any obstacles melt away.

Having journeyed to the past and to the future, now arrive at the present moment. Ask, "Where am I this Rosh HaShanah?" Witness—without judgment—feelings, images, and thoughts that arise in response to this question. Breathe in acceptance. Breathe out release. Whisper: הִנֵּנִי, "Hineini."

Slowly, when ready, open the eyes.

Write or draw.

What does הִנֵּנִי, *hineini,* mean to me?

This year, how can I show up more fully in my life?

In everything you do, you encounter sparks full of life and light,
aspiring to rise toward the heights. You help them, and they help you.

RABBI ABRAHAM ISAAC KOOK

2

Yom Kippur

The Day of Atonement

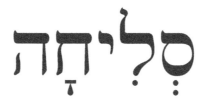

Slichah • Forgiveness

The Holy One, Blessed be God, said to Israel,
"Make an opening for repentance which is only as small as the eye of a needle,
and I will open it so wide that wagons and carriages can pass through."

MIDRASH, SHIR HASHIRIM RABBAH 5:2

HOLIDAY TRADITIONS

A Day Set Apart

- The 10 Days of Awe culminate on Yom Kippur, a day devoted entirely to repentance.

- For the 25 hours of Yom Kippur, Jews fast and refrain from wearing jewelry or leather, from washing, and from engaging in mundane activities. On Yom Kippur, a day of communal penitance, it is customary to gather at synagogue and to wear white.

- The Day of Atonement begins in the evening with a service called _Kol Nidre_ (All Vows). On this sacred evening, all Torah scrolls in the synagogue are brought out from the ark (the space in which they are housed) as Jews consider the vows which sanctify their lives.

- The prayers of Yom Kippur include multiple repetitions of the _Viddui_, a communal confession of sin. Torah reading, recitation of _Eleh Ezkerah_ (an enumeration of Jewish martyrs throughout the ages), and _Yizkor_ (a memorial service) are other powerful components of Yom Kippur observance.

- During the final _Neilah_ service, as the sun sets, the community stands before the open ark praying for a year of blessing and affirming God's sovereignty in the world.

- Yom Kippur concludes with _Havdalah_, in which a braided candle is held aloft and extinguished in a cup of wine, and a final blast of the ram's horn is sounded.

כַּוָּנוֹת הַנֶּפֶשׁ *Kavanot HaNefesh*

INTENTIONS FOR THE SOUL

Repentance and Return

On the solemn day of Yom Kippur, we shed distractions and let go of corporal needs, striving to become more like angels and to draw closer to God. The Day of Atonement opens a space in which to consider the impact of our choices and to ask ourselves: "This past year, what did I truly achieve?" "Where did I go astray?" "Which relationships need repair?" "What is most precious in my life?"

Yom Kippur challenges us to contemplate our mortality and to relinquish the masks of titles, possessions, and societal status. It is a day of intimacy with our Creator and with our souls, a day in which we pray to be inscribed in the Book of Life. This holiday is, at once, intensely personal and deeply communal. At the close of the Day of Atonement, we face the year ahead empowered, our vision clear, and our spirits cleansed.

Yom Kippur is a day of intimacy with our Creator and with our souls.

כַּוָּנוֹת הַגּוּף *Kavanot HaGuf*

INTENTIONS FOR THE BODY

Humbly Acknowledging our Humanity Before God

In our Yom Kippur yoga practice, we revere this most awesome day. This yoga practice prepares us to bow down with humility and prostrate ourselves before God. Our essential postures are the modest, submissive, and prone-facing **Child's Pose**, **Puppy Dog Pose**, and **Full Pranam Pose**. With our bodies low to the ground in partial and then full prostration, we acknowledge our humanity, our sins, and our transgressions. With bowed heads, outstretched arms, and palms facing the heavens, we crack open our hearts, praying for forgiveness and that we will be granted yet another year—inscribed in the Book of Life.

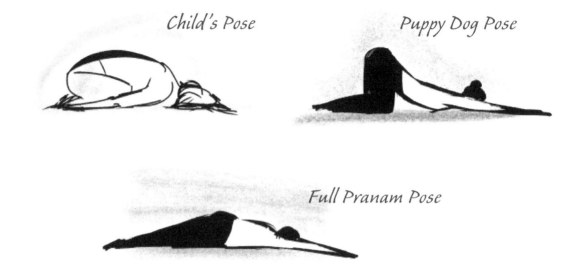

Child's Pose   *Puppy Dog Pose*

Full Pranam Pose

Child's Pose

- Come down to the ground. Sit on the lower legs, widen the knees apart with the feet touching. Relax and breathe deeply into the belly. Release the shoulders away from the ears with the arms along the sides of the body, the palms facing up. Soften the head to the floor in **Child's Pose**.
- Before God, humbly acknowledge the miracle of the life within. Breathe deeply, from the center of the body and the mind, for 5 more cycles.

Puppy Dog Pose

- Extend the arms in front and lengthen the sides of the waist. Align the hips over the knees.
- Melt the chest, forehead, and even the chin down toward the ground in **Puppy Dog Pose**. Breathe fully into the space of the torso and the intercostal muscles along the rib cage for 5 cycles.

Full Pranam Pose

- Lie facedown, fully prone on the front body, extending the legs behind and the arms forward. Flip the palms of the hands up towards the sky. Sense the yearning for God in body and soul.
- Remain here, receptive and present in **Full Pranam Pose**, for 10 breaths. Acknowledging human failing and transgression, pray for *slichah*—individual and communal forgiveness.

סְלִיחָה *Slichah* Forgiveness

Focusing on the Hebrew word above, create and expand upon your own yoga practice. Embody the themes of the holiday.

- a space for divine inspiration & practical ideas -

GUIDED MEDITATION

Find a seat for meditation.
Close the eyes.
With an alert spine, settle into stillness.
Observe the breath.
Notice any sounds. Feel the air on the skin.
Become present.

On Yom Kippur, we release all that is unnecessary and focus on our essence, our purpose, our soul. To express our intention for purity and renewal, on the Day of Atonement, we wear white.

Imagine being enveloped in a pure and cleansing light. See that light move from the crown of the head down to the feet. Breathe, gently and naturally. Sense the power and beauty of the *neshama*, the soul.

As you continue to breathe, remember one act of personal wrongdoing from the past year. Allow yourself to re-experience that moment. Breathe. Release any tension in the face. Now, offer the word: סְלִיחָה, *"Slichah,"* which means "forgiveness" or "please forgive."

In your mind's eye, turn to someone who has been hurtful in the past year. Try to gaze into their eyes. Knowing that you are safe here in this space, feel the hurt. Notice what arises in the body. Soften any tension in the face. Breathe. Again, offer the word: סְלִיחָה, *"Slichah."*

Remain in silent meditation, witnessing the experience of offering and receiving forgiveness.

Return to an awareness of the body. With gentle gestures, sweep the hands from the crown of the head to the shoulders and arms, as if brushing the body clean. Shed all that is unneeded.

Slowly, when ready, open the eyes prepared to face the year anew.

JOURNALING

Write or draw.

From whom do I need to ask forgiveness—and for what?

Whom have I not yet forgiven?
How might I take a step toward healing this connection?

Yom Kippur is not so much a Day of Atonement,
but rather a day of "at-one-ment"—
a day when we strive to be "at one" with our souls and with God.

3
Sukkot

Festival of the Harvest

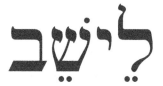

Leisheiv · To Dwell

Grant me the ability to be alone.
May it be my custom to go outdoors each day
among the trees and grasses, among all growing things;
and there may I be alone, and enter into prayer
to talk with the One to Whom I belong.

RABBI NACHMAN OF BRESLOV

HOLIDAY TRADITIONS

Abundance and Ingathering

- Sukkot is one of three annual pilgrimage festivals, celebrated since ancient times by journeying to Jerusalem.

- For seven days, Sukkot is observed by dwelling in a simple hut called a *sukkah*.

- *Sukkot* (the Hebrew word for huts) are reminiscent of the shelters in which the Jewish people lived, after the Exodus from Egypt, during their 40 years of desert wandering.

- An agricultural festival, Sukkot celebrates the bounty of the harvest. On this holiday, Jews read from the book of *Kohelet* (Ecclesiastes), which describes cycles and seasons of human life and of our natural world.

- During the seven days of Sukkot, it is traditional to eat and sleep in one's *sukkah*, inviting guests to join. In the custom of *ushpizin*, mystical visitors from ancient times are also welcomed into the sukkah.

- A central element of this holiday involves bringing together four plant species from the land of Israel: the *lulav* (palm branch), *aravah* (willow), *hadas* (myrtle), and *etrog* (citron). The bundle is admired for its beauty and scent, and then shaken in all directions, acknowledging the many forces of nature and God's surrounding presence.

- During the seventh day of Sukkot, called *Hoshannah Rabbah,* the four species are held high as participants process in seven circles or *hakafot.* On *Shemini Atzeret,* the eighth day after the start of Sukkot, prayers begin for life-giving winter rain.

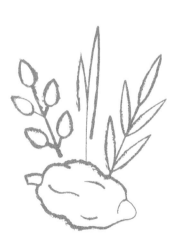

כַּוָּנוֹת הַנֶּפֶשׁ *Kavanot HaNefesh*

INTENTIONS FOR THE SOUL

Rejoicing Amidst Fragility

Sukkot encompasses the expression of fulfillment and joy alongside the awareness of our human fragility and mortality. After the intensive and elevated spiritual focus of Yom Kippur, Sukkot invites us back down to earth, to inhabit the body. We embrace physicality through the *mitzvot* (sacred acts) of building a *sukkah*, dwelling within it, and enjoying the fruits of the harvest. Our senses are awakened by the four species (palm, willow, myrtle, and citron) with their diversity of texture, shape, and fragrance. We taste delicious food, smell the autumn air, and open our eyes to the sky above, which is visible through the roof of the *sukkah*. Even with its spirit of celebration, Sukkot calls our attention to the transient nature of all life. For a *sukkah* cannot protect us from the rain or the approaching chill of winter.

Sukkot invites us back down to earth, to inhabit the body.

כַּוָּנוֹת הַגּוּף *Kavanot HaGuf*

INTENTIONS FOR THE BODY

Opening Our Hearts, Fully Vulnerable and Alive

In our Sukkot yoga practice, we embody the cycle of life and the agricultural year. This practice emphasizes gratitude and thanksgiving for the bounty of the season. Our essential postures are the uplifting, stimulating, and energizing **Bridge Pose**, **Wheel Pose**, and **Locust Pose**. These circular, arching poses mirror the arc of life's season and the ongoing cycles found in nature and the cosmos. We rise up, in body and soul, opening at the heart center, challenging the flexibility of our spine and our spirit, embracing the experience of being fully vulnerable and alive.

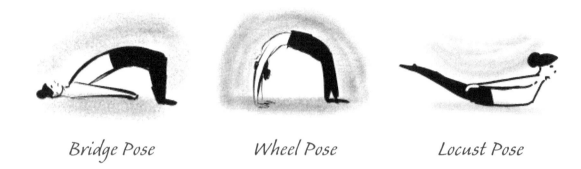

Bridge Pose   *Wheel Pose*   *Locust Pose*

Bridge Pose

- Lying on the back, bend the knees and place the feet on the floor, hip distance apart. Press down through the feet, lifting and elevating the pelvis. Snuggle the arms and shoulder blades inward, interlacing the fingers beneath the lower back.

- Expand the belly and chest into **Bridge Pose**. Feel the energy, strength, and vitality throughout the hip and buttock muscles. As breath moves in and out, acknowledge the cycles and celebrations of life.

- Continue to lift the chest. Expand and feel the spaciousness around the heart and lungs. Remain in **Bridge Pose** for 5 breaths. Roll down sequentially through the upper, middle, and lower back, releasing to the ground. Widen the feet apart and rest the knees together. Repeat this pose 1-3 times.

Wheel Pose

- Rotate the elbows back and up, and place the hands with the palms down by the ears. Hug the elbows in and lift the chest backward. Press into the palms and extend the arms with strength and vigor.

- Lift the hips and buttocks off the ground, drawing the tailbone toward the knees, lengthening the lower back up and into **Wheel Pose**.

- Stretch open the front body and strengthen the back body. Feel the vigor and vibration of life in the full bounty of this pose. Hold for 3-5 cycles of breath.

- Release and rest.

לֵישֵׁב *Leisheiv* To Dwell

Focusing on the Hebrew word above, create and expand upon your own yoga practice. Embody the themes of the holiday.

- a space for divine inspiration & practical ideas -

Locust Pose

- Lie on the belly and press the toes into the floor, engaging the legs. Reach back with the toes, and rotate the inner thighs inward and upward to broaden and lengthen the lower back.
- Engage the abdominal core muscles extending the spine. Lift the chest, arms, and legs up and back into **Locust Pose**. Rise up with energy in the pose for 3-5 breaths. Release and rest in a prone position, facing the ground.
- Experience gratitude for the shelter that the body provides for the soul, and for the potential of renewal. Find joy in this moment. Say to yourself, *"Leisheiv"* (to dwell).

GUIDED MEDITATION

Find a seat for meditation.*
Close the eyes.
With an alert spine, settle into stillness.
Observe the breath.
Notice any sounds. Feel the air on the skin.
Become present.

Firmly planted on the "sits" bones with the spine erect, visualize the body as a *sukkah*. Our physical form is beautiful, a dwelling for celebration.

Each of the four species of Sukkot calls attention to the physical self: the spine (the palm branch), the heart (the etrog), the lips (the willow), the eyes (the myrtle). Breathe. Allow the spine to sway. Feel the beating heart. Invite the lips to come to a smile. Imagine the eyes shining behind closed lids.

Honor the magnificent construction of the body, its shape and form. Offer aloud the word: לֵישֵׁב, *"Leisheiv."* It is a blessing to be alive, to be surrounded by community, to be connected to this body and to this earth. Breathe in and out. Feel the air on the skin. Listen.

Draw attention to the crown of the head, releasing any tension in the face or scalp. Now, shift the focus to that which is beyond the head—to the roof of the *sukkah* in which you dwell. Open to an awareness of the sky, the stars, the cosmos. Breathe.

Return and focus on our shared connection to this earth and to the dwelling place of the body—strong and fragile, joyful and temporary. Once again, offer the word: לֵישֵׁב, *"Leisheiv."*

Slowly, when ready, open the eyes.

*Because it is Sukkot, you may wish to sit outdoors or in a Sukkah.

JOURNALING

Write or draw.

Today, what is my foundation? What shelters me?

This year, where and how do I want לֵישֵׁב, *leisheiv* (to dwell)?

This too shall pass.

SAYING FROM AN ANCIENT JEWISH FOLKTALE

4

Simchat Torah

The Joy of Torah

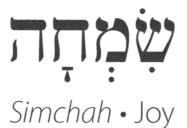

שִׂמְחָה

Simchah · Joy

Praise God with timbrels and dance.

PSALM 149:3

HOLIDAY TRADITIONS

The Neverending Cycle of Torah

- Falling immediately after the eight-day holiday of Sukkot, Simchat Torah marks the renewal of the annual cycle of weekly Torah reading.

- On Simchat Torah, Jews gather at synagogue, where the last verses of the book of Deuteronomy are chanted—followed immediately by the opening verses of the book of Genesis. This initiates the beginning of the year's Torah reading cycle.

- During the evening that opens this holiday, each synagogue's Torah scrolls are removed from the ark (the space in which they are housed) with singing and dancing in seven *hakafot* (circles). As a part of the celebration, dancing often overflows outdoors onto the street.

- Offering the blessings before and after the reading of Torah is a special honor granted on this holiday.

- During Simchat Torah celebrations in some communities, a Torah scroll is unrolled, in its entirety, for all to see.

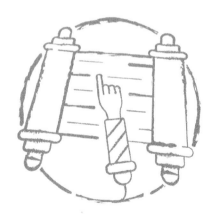

כַּוָּנוֹת הַנֶּפֶשׁ *Kavanot HaNefesh*

INTENTIONS FOR THE SOUL

Exulting in Our Sacred Scroll

With the literal meaning "Joy of Torah", Simchat Torah represents a cathartic culmination of the High Holy Days season. Bursting with joyful, communal celebration. Simchat Torah coincides with the change of seasons in Israel and, thus, prayers for rain. Water, like Torah, provides life-giving sustenance. As we bridge from the story of Moses' death (in the last verses of Torah) to that of the world's creation (described in Torah's opening verses), we affirm the cycles of renewal that define Jewish time. Carrying and dancing with a sacred Torah scroll is a symbol of Jewish pride and hope in the future. Simchat Torah expresses our commitment to live by the rules of Torah and to make them real in our lives.

Carrying and dancing with a sacred Torah scroll is a symbol of Jewish pride and hope in the future.

כַּוָּנוֹת הַגּוּף *Kavanot HaGuf*

INTENTIONS FOR THE BODY

Invigorating Joy and Love for Torah and God

In our Simchat Torah yoga practice, we acknowledge and celebrate the end and the beginning of the Torah reading cycle. This yoga practice reinvigorates our commitment to and love of Torah and God. Our essential postures are the expansive, ecstatic **Camel Pose** and the alert, upright **Hero Pose**. Warming up with **Cow and Cat Poses** prepares the spine to stretch into a backbend.

Camel Pose facilitates the exhilaration which comes from being wide open at the heart and throat. In this pose, we might imagine the body opening and unraveling spaciously as would a Torah scroll. In the vertical seat of **Hero Pose**, we come to an erect spine—recharged and ready to begin anew.

תְּנוּעוֹת חִיוּנִיּוֹת   *T'nu'ot Chiyuniyot*

ESSENTIAL POSES

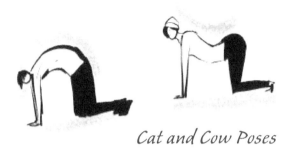

Cat and Cow Poses

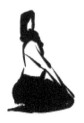

Camel Pose

Hero Pose

Cat and Cow Pose

- Warm up the body by coming onto all fours, with the hips stacked over the knees and the shoulders over the wrists.

- With straight arms, exhale, rounding the upper back and spreading shoulder blades apart. Lengthen and tone the tailbone downward, gazing toward the navel in **Cat Pose**. Inhale and draw the shoulder blades together. Dropping the belly and arching the spine, look upward and outward in **Cow Pose**. Repeat 3-5 times.

Camel Pose

- With the feet hip width apart, rise to a kneeling position on the shins and knees. Press the pelvis over the knees, with the belly toning in and the tailbone lengthening down.

- Draw the shoulder blades back, opening the chest. Place the hands on the lower back or grasp the heels. Lengthen the neck and gently release the head back.

- Remain in **Camel Pose** for 5 cycles of breath. Feel expansion across the throat and the heart. Experience the joy, energy, and exhilaration of dropping back.

Hero pose

- Come to a seat on the lower legs, moving the feet and calves to the outside of the hips with the knees touching in **Hero Pose**. As a modified variation, place a block or cushion under the seat and root the tailbone down into the prop.

- Press the tops of the feet into the floor, tone the front ribs in, and relax the neck, sitting upright and alert. Receive the bright energy of the pose and allow a smile to emanate from your face and spread throughout your entire being. Say to yourself, *"Simchah"* (joy).

שִׂמְחָה *Simchah* Joy

*Focusing on the Hebrew word above, create and expand upon
your own yoga practice. Embody the themes of the holiday.*

- a space for divine inspiration & practical ideas -

GUIDED MEDITATION

Find a seat for meditation.
Close the eyes.
With an alert spine, settle into stillness.
Observe the breath.
Notice any sounds. Feel the air on the skin.
Become present.

With each breath, visualize oxygen filling the lungs, enlivening the body. Experience breath as a source of expansive joy. Continue to breathe. Imagining the oxygenated blood circulating throughout the body. Notice any sensations that arise. Wiggle the fingers and toes. Gently roll the head, releasing any tension in the face and shoulders.

With an inhalation, imagine the sound שִׂם *sim*, and with an exhale, imagine the sound חָה *chah*. Continue for a few cycles of breath.

Invite a smile to the face, not just with the lips but with each muscle of the forehead, eyes, and cheeks. Allow the smile and joy to permeate into the heart center and expand throughout the entire body. Just as Torah scrolls are carried high on Simchat Torah, envision being surrounded and lifted by a circle of love, joy, and support.

Repeat the word: שִׂמְחָה *"Simchah."*

Slowly, when ready, open the eyes and see the world with joy.

Write or draw.

What brings me שִׂמְחָה. *simchah* (joy)?

How might I bring an intention for joy more fully into my life?

She is a tree of life to those who grasp her,
bringing happiness to all who hold her tight.

PROVERBS 3:18

5
Hanukkah

The Festival
of Lights

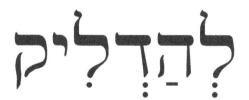

L'hadlik · To Ignite

You cannot chase darkness with a stick.
You must strike a match.

JEWISH PROVERB

מְסוֹרֶת הֶחָג *Masoret HeChag*

HOLIDAY TRADITIONS

A Story of Miracles and Might

- The eight-day holiday of Hanukkah commemorates the period in Jewish history when Antiochus and the Assyrian-Greeks took over and desecrated the Temple in Jerusalem, punishing Jews who remained loyal to their tradition.

- A small group, led by Judah Maccabee, attacked the Syrian-Greek army. Miraculously, the Maccabees emerged victorious, taking back and rededicating the Temple. Thus, the Hebrew word *Hanukkah* means dedication.

- Only one cruse of oil remained to light the Temple's *menorah* (a sacred candelabrum), but the oil lasted—enabling the *menorah's* light to burn for eight days. On Hanukkah, Jews celebrate this ancient miracle of the oil by enjoying fried treats like *latkes* (potato pancakes).

- Games are played using a *dreidel* (spinning top). Written on each side of the *dreidel* are the Hebrew letters *nun, gimmel, hey, shin,* which stand for *Nes Gadol Haya Sham* ("A great miracle happened there").

- On Hanukkah, each household's menorah (also called a *hanukkiyah*) is placed in the window for all to see.

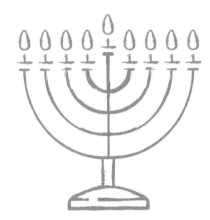

כַּוָּנוֹת הַנֶּפֶשׁ *Kavanot HaNefesh*

INTENTIONS FOR THE SOUL

The Courage to Kindle Flame

Hanukkah inspires us to act with courage and to bring light to dark places. In the short, cold days of winter, Hanukkah reminds us that we can move through challenges by accessing strength and vision. When the Assyrian-Greeks were in power, many chose to assimilate, abandoning Judaism for Greek culture and beliefs. Yet others, like Judah Maccabee and his band of warriors, chose to fight back. Hanukkah inspires us to stand in our truth no matter what others may say or dictate. Times of darkness can spur us to connect with our inner flame—the light and energy of the body. Yet, to do so, we need *ruach* (spirit or wind). Just as fire needs oxygen to burn brightly, we need breath and spirit to access our power.

Hanukkah inspires us to stand in our truth no matter what others may say or dictate.

כַּוָּנוֹת הַגּוּף *Kavanot HaGuf*

INTENTIONS FOR THE BODY

Igniting Sparks of Courage, Justice, and Truth

Our Hanukkah yoga practice, with strong and sustained poses, builds heat and energy in the body and mind. This heat stimulates and burns off stagnation and lethargy, creating the potential for transformation. The essential postures are the grounding, steadfast, and balanced **Warrior I**, **Warrior II**, and **Warrior III Poses**. By engaging and activating our feet, legs, hips, arms, and abdominal muscles, we ignite a flame that moves from the outside in, from body to soul, directing us toward bravery, justice, and truth. Let's burn off doubt and fear as we deepen our breath and step into the steady strength and courage of a Maccabee warrior.

ESSENTIAL POSES

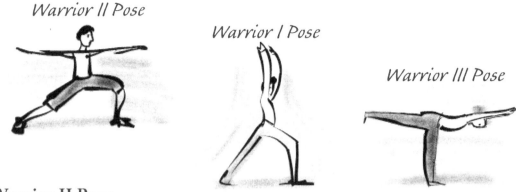

Warrior II Pose

Warrior I Pose

Warrior III Pose

Warrior II Pose

- Step the legs approximately 3 feet apart. Rotate the right (front) foot, knee, and hip outward, bending the knee into a 90-degree angle. Pivot the left (back) foot and hip inward. Commit to grounding and toning the feet and legs.

- Keep the torso over the pelvis. Actively extend the right arm forward and the left arm back, at shoulder height and parallel to the floor. Gently tone the belly and draw the front ribs in. Gaze over the right fingers in **Warrior II Pose**. Be steady and focused. Inhale, breathing in strength; exhale, breathing out presence, for 5 breaths.

- Pivot the feet and hips to reorient, and repeat **Warrior II** sequence on the other side.

Warrior I Pose

- Start by standing with the feet parallel at the front of the mat. Step the right leg back 3 feet, internally rotating the hips. Firmly root through the feet and legs. Align the left knee over the left heel, bending the knee into a 90-degree angle.

- Square the hips and shoulders forward. Lift the front of the pelvis. Lengthen the tailbone.

- Reach the arms upward, shoulder width apart. Gaze forward, elongating the neck. Hold **Warrior I Pose** for 5 breaths.

Warrior III Pose

- From **Warrior I Pose**, transition the weight forward to balance on the front leg. Square the front hip, and internally rotate the back hip and leg. Prepare to balance, lifting the back leg into the air, level at hip height. Flex the toes.

לְהַדְלִיק *L'hadlik* To Ignite

Focusing on the Hebrew word above, create and expand upon your own yoga practice. Embody the themes of the holiday.

- a space for divine inspiration & practical ideas -

- Extend the chest and heart forward. Steady the gaze. With focused attention, tone the limbs in toward the midline of the body and simultaneously relax the shoulders and extend the arms out in **Warrior III Pose**. Remain in this position for 5 breaths.

- Release and recover, stepping the right foot to meet the left. Stand tall for a moment.

- Now, repeat **Warrior I to Warrior III sequence** on the other side. Through these bold poses, acknowledge the right to stand up and to ignite—*l'hadlik*—a flame for vision, truth, and justice.

Find a seat for meditation.
Close the eyes.
With an alert spine, settle into stillness.
Observe the breath.
Notice any sounds. Feel the air on the skin.
Become present.

For those meditating before a lit *hanukkiah*, integrate the prompts offered in bold.

The Hanukkah candles are not to be used for any purpose other than to celebrate the miracle of the oil, the miracle of human courage. We are not to work as they burn. Take these moments to be still and to witness the energy and sensations of the body, the movement of the mind.

Relax your eyes, and with a steady gaze, observe the flames of the *hanukkiah*. What do you see? What do you feel? Take in the miracle of the light.

Imagine the body as a candle: the spine—the wick at the center. Our muscles, sinews and skin—the wax surrounding that wick. With light and heat, wax melts and takes on new forms; so too can the body become supple and transform.

With eyes closed, bring awareness to each body part, beginning at the feet and moving up the legs and along the spine to the crown of the head. Notice feelings of "light" (spaciousness, vibrancy, energy). Breathe into those spaces.

Whisper the word: לְהַדְלִיק, "*L'hadlik.*"

Inhale. Feel warm and bright. Exhale. Feel cool and dark. Celebrate the interplay of energies—shadowy darkness and energized light. Acknowledge the depth of winter's night which gives meaning to Hanukkah's flame. Sense the light within.

Once again, whisper the word: לְהַדְלִיק, "*L'hadlik.*"

Slowly, when ready, open the eyes.

For a few more cycles of breath, witness the dancing flames of the menorah.*

**Some may wish to remain present, observing the candle flames until the very last one has flickered out.*

JOURNALING

Write or draw.

For what do I need courage and strength?

What ignites my energy, imagination, and hope?

Not by might. Not by power, but by My spirit—said the God of Hosts.

ZECHARIA 4:6

6

Tu B'Shevat

The Birthday of the Trees

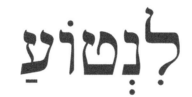

Linto'ah • To Plant

A human being is likened to a tree of the field.

COMMENTARY ON DEUTERONOMY 20:19

HOLIDAY TRADITIONS

A Celebration of Root, Trunk, Branch, and Blossom

- Tu B'Shevat means the 15th of the Hebrew month *Shevat*. In the land of Israel, Tu B'Shevat arrives in early spring when most of the winter rains have fallen, and the almond trees have begun to bloom.

- During ancient times, the New Year of the Trees served a fiscal and agricultural purpose, enabling farmers to determine the age of a tree in order to tithe and harvest its fruit.

- In modern times, the observance of Tu B'Shevat has continued to evolve, taking on new relevance. Tree planting is central to the vitality of the State of Israel. Tree and forest preservation is essential to the well-being of our planet.

- The New Year of the Trees has mystical elements, as well. In 16th-century Tsfat in Northern Israel, the Kabbalists created a Tu B'Shevat seder. At such a seder, four cups of wine or grape juice are enjoyed. The first cup is white, with increasing amounts of crimson or purple grape juice added to the second, third, and fourth cups—symbolizing the growing bounty and color of spring. At a Tu B'Shevat seder, the fruits of the land of Israel are consumed, with the qualities of these fruits being likened to the facets of the human soul.

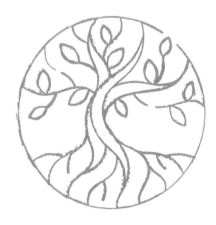

כַּוָּנוֹת הַנֶּפֶשׁ *Kavanot HaNefesh*

INTENTIONS FOR THE SOUL

Rise from Rest to Blossom and Balance

Tu B'Shevat celebrates the interplay between winter hibernation and the rebirth of spring. The New Year of the Trees invites us to anchor into our roots—our families and friends, our communities, and the earth which sustains us. Digging deep and soaking up the winter rain enlivens us to stretch upward, blossoming toward the sky. On Tu B'Shevat, we acknowledge the holy, hidden, and mysterious potential in all physical reality: the dormant seed, the green sprout, the fresh blossom, the first fruit of the season. Tu B'Shevat affirms our precious bond with the land of Israel and with all creation. As we sense the early stirrings of spring, we remember the necessity of planting ourselves in soil which nourishes our growth.

Digging deep and soaking up the winter rain enlivens us to stretch upward, blossoming toward the sky.

כַּוָּנוֹת הַגּוּף *Kavanot HaGuf*

INTENTIONS FOR THE BODY

Embracing the Renewal of Spring

In our Tu B'Shevat yoga practice, we explore the juxtaposition of earth and sky, stability and flexibility, gravity and levity, hibernation and awakening. The essential postures are the hip-opening **Garland** and **Tree Poses** in which we stretch our hips, release habitual tension and stagnation, and awaken to our potential. This yoga practice lowers us toward the nourishing earth with **Garland Pose** through which we connect to the element of water and of saturating winter rains, enabling flow, fluidity, and creativity. In **Tree Pose**, we press our feet and roots down into the earth, expanding our limbs and trunk upright toward the sun. Through these postures, we embrace the promise and renewal of spring.

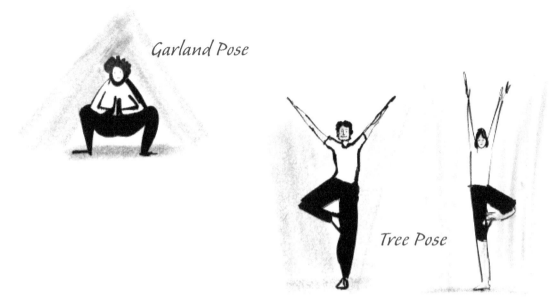

Garland Pose

Tree Pose

Garland Pose

- Step the legs wider than hip-width apart. Turn the heels slightly inward and the toes outward. Bend and track the knees over the feet, lower the tailbone, and squat the hips toward the earth.
- Bring the hands together in front of the heart, broadening at the collarbone. Wiggle, and press the elbows against the inner thighs.
- Lift and lengthen the spine away from the ground, gently toning the pelvic floor muscles. Marinate in **Garland Pose** for 5 cycles of breath. Fold into a forward bend to recover, and release to rise.

Tree Pose

- Stand upright with both feet rooted. Then, lift the left foot, bend the knee, and shift the weight onto the right foot. Turn the left knee and hip out, pressing the foot against the right leg either at the thigh, shin, or ankle.
- Extend both arms actively skyward, dropping the shoulders away from the ears. Engage the abdominal core muscles. Imagine a favorite tree blooming after winter, and set your sights on a creative aspiration for the coming spring.
- Balance with a steady, soft gaze in **Tree Pose** for 5 cycles of breath.
- Release the pose, planting both feet firmly into the ground, Pause, and repeat the sequence leading to **Tree Pose** on the other side. Envision sowing and cultivating seeds of renewal for spring—*linto'ah*.

לִנְטוֹעַ *Linto'ah* To Plant

Focusing on the Hebrew word above, create and expand upon
your own yoga practice. Embody the themes of the holiday.

- a space for divine inspiration & practical ideas -

Find a seat for meditation.
Close the eyes.
With an alert spine, settle into stillness.
Observe the breath.
Notice any sounds. Feel the air on the skin.
Become present.

Consider the soil in which roots are planted. With eyes closed, envision the fertile, cool earth. Breathe in and breathe out. Whisper the word: לִנְטוֹעַ, *"Linto'ah."* Imagine roots deepening and spreading so as to draw in sustenance.

Consider that which sustains and nourishes life. Bless those elements.

Now, raise up an aspiration for this spring. In the mind's eye, see a sapling extending toward the sun. Imagine achieving this dream. Envision this new blossom of springtime hope ripening into a first fruit. Once again, offer the word: לִנְטוֹעַ, *"Linto'ah."*

Slowly, when ready, open the eyes.

JOURNALING

Write or draw.

What seeds do I want לִנְטוֹעַ, *linto'ah* (to plant) this winter?

How do I imagine myself blooming this spring?

*Just as I found the world full of carob trees
planted by my parents and grandparents,
so I will plant for my children.*

TALMUD, TA'ANIT 23A

7

Purim

Chance, Masks, and Merriment

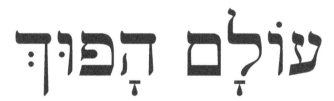

Olam Hafuch
A World Turned Upside Down

*And so, on the 13th day of the 12th month—that is, the month of Adar—
when the king's command and decree were to be carried out,
the very day on which the enemies of the Jews had expected to overpower them,
the opposite happened...*

MEGILLAT ESTHER 9:1

HOLIDAY TRADITIONS

Laughter and Unexpected Salvation

- Purim is celebrated by listening to *Megillat Esther* (The Scroll of Esther), which contains a story of unexpected Jewish survival.

- After the destruction of the first Temple, Jews were exiled to Persia, where the king's advisor, Haman, sought to annihilate them. Yet, just in time, Esther and her uncle Mordechai intervened to save their people.

- On Purim, Jews dress up in costume, indulge in drinking alcohol, and enjoy a festive holiday meal with sweets such as *hamentashen* (triangle cookies made in the shape of Haman's hat). Purim customs include giving gifts of food, called *mishlo'ach manot*, to friends, and offering *tzedakah* (charity) to those in need.

- During the reading of *Megillat Esther*, with each recitation of Haman's name, *groggers* (noisemakers) are sounded. This symbolizes Jewish commitment to "remember to forget" all who seek their destruction.

- Purim falls on the 14th of *Adar*, the Hebrew month that increases joy.

- Yet, even with its revelry, Purim carries a sober message about Jewish vulnerability and the presence of evil in this world. In *Megillat Esther,* salvation arrives—not through Divine intervention but through human hands. In fact, in the entire Scroll of Esther, God's name is hidden, not mentioned even once.

כַּוָּנוֹת הַנֶּפֶשׁ *Kavanot HaNefesh*

INTENTIONS FOR THE SOUL

Challenging Our Expectations

Megillat Esther unfolds against the lavish and precarious backdrop of the ancient Persian royal court. This holiday of costumes and masks draws our attention to hidden possibilities, reminding us that there is more to ourselves (and to others) than meets the eye. In *Megillat Esther*, our assumptions are turned upside down: The king is a buffoon while the ingenue is a courageous heroine. The day on which the Jewish people were to be destroyed becomes the day of their salvation. Purim reminds us that, in our ever-changing, unpredictable world, we can counter fear with *chutzpah* (audacious confidence). Just as Esther stepped forward to save her people, we too can move from vulnerability to strength, experiencing a reversal of expectations and newfound outcomes.

*In Megillat Esther,
 our assumptions are turned upside down.*

כַּוָּנוֹת הַגּוּף *Kavanot HaGuf*

INTENTIONS FOR THE BODY

Facing Fear and Vulnerability with Perspective

In our Purim yoga practice, we turn ourselves upside down with the essential, inverted postures of **Downward Facing Dog**, **Headstand**, **Shoulderstand**, and **Plough**. The benefits of inversions are many. Physically, we activate our core strength, aligning and toning the muscles along our entire spine. We stimulate and reverse the blood flow to all our major organs. Spiritually, being upside down requires us to see our situation anew. Inversions also uncover our vulnerability, our fear of falling. Lowering our heads and lifting our feet and tail bones up, we turn our orientation inward. In the headstand pose, with the crown of the head on the ground and our feet reaching skyward, everything looks vice versa. These poses may appear a bit precarious or even absurd to an onlooker. Thus, it is with caution and exuberance that we challenge ourselves to invert and, as we do so, to reveal a bold new reality.

תְּנוּעוֹת חִיּוּנִיּוֹת *T'nu'ot Chiyuniyot*
ESSENTIAL POSES

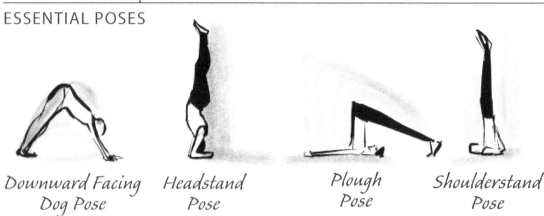

Downward Facing Dog Pose   Headstand Pose   Plough Pose   Shoulderstand Pose

Downward Facing Dog Pose

- From all fours on hands and knees, root the wrists under the shoulders and the knees under the hips; spread the fingers. Press the toes into the ground and lift the pelvis, extending back through the legs.
- Push into the hands, lengthening up through the arms and the sides of the waist. Draw the front ribs inward.
- Release the head and neck to dangle between the arms. Gaze toward the navel. Breathe for 5 cycles in **Downward Facing Dog Pose**.

Headstand Pose

(Note: This pose may be practiced against a wall for extra support.)

- Begin on hands and knees. Lower the forearms to the floor. Interlace the fingers and press down on the outer edge of the wrists.
- Place the crown of the head into the cradle of the hands. Pressing the forearms down, draw the front ribs in, and activate the abdominal core. Slowly walk the feet closer to the head. Bending the knees, carefully lift the legs up into **Headstand Pose**.
- Straighten the legs up towards the sky, lifting the shoulders away from the ears. Keep the neck steady. Breathe rhythmically for 5-10 cycles. Adapt and adjust to being upside down. Simultaneously gaze with an inward and outward focus.
- Gently come out of the pose. Rest and recover in the **Child's Pose** (see page 101 in the Yoga Appendix) for several breaths, integrating the experience of inversion.

Plough Pose

- Prepare by lying on the back in a supine, face-upward position, hugging the knees into the chest.

YOUR YOGA SEQUENCE

עוֹלָם הָפוּךְ *Olam Hafuch* A World Turned Upside Down

*Focusing on the Hebrew words above, create and expand upon
your own yoga practice. Embody the themes of the holiday.*

- a space for divine inspiration & practical ideas -

- Pressing your hands into the floor, playfully rock and roll on the spine a few times, forward and backward, engaging the abdominal core and lifting the legs up into the air.
- Bring the hips over the shoulders and the toes over the head to the floor. Lift the chin and press the forearms down in **Plough Pose**. Breathe for 5 cycles.

Shoulderstand Pose

- From the **Plough Pose**, draw the shoulders in and upper arms under the back. Walk the hands up to press along each side of the spine, stacking the hips above the shoulders.
- Extend the legs straight up, spreading through the toes and elevating the hips toward the sky, to come into **Shoulderstand Pose**.
- With the chin lifted and the gaze steady towards the navel, maintain a curve at the back of the neck. Breathe for 5 cycles.
- Mindfully roll down through the spine, release, rest, and recover.

GUIDED MEDITATION

Find a seat for meditation.
Close the eyes.
With an alert spine, settle into stillness.
Observe the breath.
Notice any sounds. Feel the air on the skin.
Become present.

Bring awareness to the seat at the pelvis and legs. Now, shift the focus to just above the crown of the head. Bring presence to the upper and lower spheres, the front and back planes, the left and right sides, the physical and spiritual realms. Experience wholeness. Each person is an entire world. Each human being is a unique life force, containing channels that can ignite infinite connections and bring about limitless outcomes.

Gently cover the eyes with the palms of the hands. Continue to breathe in and out. Now, lower the hands to rest on the thighs. Turn one palm up and the other down. Offer the words: עוֹלָם הָפוּךְ, *"Olam hafuch."*

Now, invert each palm from its present position and again offer the words: עוֹלָם הָפוּךְ, *"Olam hafuch."* Repeat this hand sequence a few more times. Acknowledge any way in which life feels simultaneously precarious but stable, absurd but real. Hold space for all to be true. Breathe. Allow the corners of the lips and eyes to turn upward into a smile. Breathe.

Slowly, when ready, open the eyes.

JOURNALING

Write or draw.

What new perspective can I share with the world?

How might I experience the world and myself differently?

Remember, things can change from the very worst to the very best...
in the blink of an eye.

RABBI NACHMAN OF BRESLOV

8

Passover

The Story
of Freedom

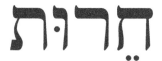

Heirut • Freedom

The Israelites went into the sea on dry ground,
the waters forming a wall for them
on their right and on their left.

EXODUS 14:22

HOLIDAY TRADITIONS

Reliving the Exodus from Egypt

- Passover (Pesach) is one of three annual pilgrimage festivals, celebrated since ancient times by journeying to Jerusalem.

- Through the holiday of Passover, Jews relive the experience of their liberation from slavery through the Exodus from Egypt.

- To prepare for this early spring holiday, Jews cleanse their homes of *hametz* (leavened products) and refrain from eating them for the eight days of Passover.

- The holiday begins in the evening with a festive meal called a *seder* (order). The Haggadah (the book of readings for the *seder* service) is read during the *seder* and retells the story of the departure from Egypt, when the angel of death passed over the homes of the soon-to-be liberated Hebrew slaves.

- The Passover *seder* meal centers around six core symbols: *matzah* (unleavened bread), *maror* (bitter herbs), *haroset* (sweet fruit paste), *z'roah* (a shank bone), *karpas* (greens, such as parsley), *hazaret* (a second bitter herb, usually lettuce), and *beitza* (a roasted egg).

- Also on the table are three pieces of covered *matzah*; salt water in which to dip the parsley; four cups of wine, consumed over the course of the seder meal; and Elijah's cup, a fifth cup of wine symbolizing redemption).

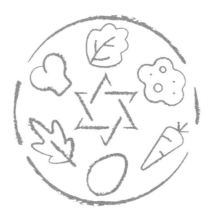

כַּוָּנוֹת הַנֶּפֶשׁ *Kavanot HaNefesh*

INTENTIONS FOR THE SOUL

Cleansing, Freedom, and Rebirth

On Passover, as we remember our people's journey to freedom, we open ourselves to the possibility of human liberation from all forces, structures, and habits which might enslave. By observing this holiday, we cleanse ourselves of constriction, inertia, and apathy. Spring awakens us to leave *Mitzrayim* (Egypt), the narrow place, and to create space for growth and renewal. Transformation from slavery to freedom requires a leap of faith. In order to leave Egypt, we dove into the Red Sea, splitting it open, creating a passageway to a new life. Today, how might we liberate ourselves or others from narrowness? On Passover, we stretch to embrace the unknown, asking courageous questions, experiencing new possibilities and unexpected expansion.

Transformation from slavery to freedom requires a leap of faith.

כַּוָּנוֹת הַגּוּף *Kavanot HaGuf*

INTENTIONS FOR THE BODY

Leaping with Faith Towards Freedom

In our Passover yoga practice, we challenge ourselves to open the hip and hamstring muscles. These essential postures allow us to confront our own "narrow places" of restriction—*Mitzrayim* (Egypt)—in the body. We warm our hamstring muscles in **Lunge Pose**, deepening into the possibility of **Full Split Pose**, then widening into **Straddle Pose**. We coax ourselves out of limitation, stretching beyond tight bodies and hesitant minds. Striving to open beyond our comfort zone, we glimpse a greater range of motion in the body and journey toward the potential for more space and freedom. With hope, persistence and a leap of faith, we may find that expansion and liberation are within reach.

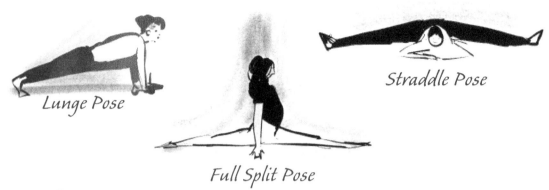

Lunge Pose

Full Split Pose

Straddle Pose

Lunge Pose

- From all fours, step the right foot forward into **Lunge Pose**. Track the right (front) knee over the foot. Lengthen the tailbone back. With the fingers on the floor, repeatedly exhale, and lower the left (back) knee to the floor. Then, inhale and re-extend the leg long and strong. Repeat 5 times.
- Straightening the front leg, lower the back knee to the floor and ease into a modified split. Release the shoulders away from the ears, and breathe for 5 cycles.

Split Pose

- Gradually slide the left knee back and the right leg forward to the point at which you can straighten the front leg. Wriggle your heel forward and draw the front hip back. Work to internally rotate both legs and lower the hips toward the ground. Continuing to breathe deeply. Remain in **Split Pose** for 3-5 cycles of breath.
- Come to an edge of sensation that is challenging and manageable. Honor and accept the limitations and restrictions of the body while affirming the fortitude of the spirit to continue. Keep the hands on the ground or, if possible, challenge yourself to extend the arms upward.
- Carefully release back, and rest in **Child's Pose** (see page 101 in the Yoga Appendix).
- Now, switch sides with the left leg forward in **Lunge Pose** and repeat the sequence into the modified or possibly **Full Split** pose.

Straddle Pose

- Sitting on the floor, extend and open the legs wide apart. Keep the pelvis rooted toward the ground. Engage and tone the leg muscles. Flex the heels so the knees and toes point upward.

חֵרוּת *Heirut* Freedom

*Focusing on the Hebrew word above, create and expand upon
your own yoga practice. Embody the themes of the holiday.*

- a space for divine inspiration & practical ideas -

- Inhale and lengthen the spine. Exhale to lower the torso toward the floor, trying not to round the back, coming into **Straddle Pose**. Remain in this pose for 5 cycles of breath.
- Recover, and feel the transformative *heirut* (freedom), after this expansive stretch.

GUIDED MEDITATION

Find a seat for meditation.
Close the eyes.
With an alert spine, settle into stillness.
Observe the breath.
Notice any sounds. Feel the air on the skin.
Become present.

Bring awareness to the seat. Witness, without judgment, any sensations in the hips and legs.

What has been released or opened through this practice? Where might even more spaciousness be? With an in breath and an exhale, invite that freedom.

Remain here for a few cycles of breath, welcoming the oxygen of hope, faith, courage, and transformation to circulate throughout the body and mind.

Offer the word: חֵרוּת, *"Heirut."* Take time for each breath. Notice. Release. Repeat: חֵרוּת, *"Heirut."*

Slowly, when ready, open the eyes.

Write or draw.

When is a time in my life that I have embraced חֵרוּת, *heirut* (freedom)?

What new חֵרוּת, *heirut* (freedom) am I seeking in the coming months—for myself and for others?

Thus says Adonai, the God of the Hebrews:
"Let My people go!"

EXODUS 9:13

9

Counting
of the Omer

From Freedom to Revelation

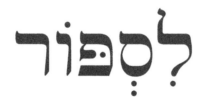

Lispor • To Count

*The world stands upon three things:
on Torah, on prayer, and on acts of loving kindness.*

PIRKE AVOT, THE ETHICS OF THE FATHERS 1:2

HOLIDAY TRADITIONS

Counting Time from Liberation to Covenant

- The Counting of the Omer begins on the eve of the second day of Passover and continues for seven weeks. An *omer* refers to a sheaf of barley, the first harvest of spring that was brought to the Temple in ancient times.

- In modern observance, the Omer is counted each night with a special blessing.

- The 49 days of the Omer mark a period of introspection. During the Counting of the Omer, some Jews refrain from having weddings, from getting haircuts, and from listening to joyful music.

- Lag BaOmer, the 33rd day of the Omer (a 24-hour festive break from solemnity), is celebrated with outdoor games, bonfires, haircuts and weddings.

- Through a mystical lens, each week of the Omer affords the opportunity to focus on a specific personal attribute: kindness, discipline, beauty, fortitude, humility, bonding, and leadership. Each quality relates to one of the seven *sephirot* (lower emanations) of the Divine.

- Seven weeks of Omer counting lead to the holiday of Shavuot, preparing the individual and the Jewish community to celebrate receiving Torah at Sinai.

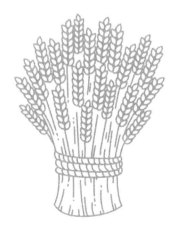

כַּוָנוֹת הַנֶפֶשׁ *Kavanot HaNefesh*

INTENTIONS FOR THE SOUL

Deepening Awareness, Finding Balance, Seeking Purpose

Counting the Omer reminds us to slow down and pay attention, to count each day, and to make each day count. Because the Omer acts as a bridge between Passover and Shavuot, this 49-day period teaches that freedom alone is not enough. Our Passover liberation journey is merely a portal, a gateway to Shavuot and to Mount Sinai where we found purpose through covenant with God. Counting the Omer inspires us to mirror the divine by finding balance between kindness, discipline, beauty, fortitude, humility, bonding, and leadership. By focusing on a single attribute for each week of the Omer, we allow these qualities to imbue our lives with sanctity. Yet, if any of them become exaggerated or are ignored, imbalance arises. In counting the Omer, we ask: How might I express each of these attributes so as to bring greater harmony to my own life and to the world? By approaching this seven-week period with intention, awareness, and effort, we arrive at the holiday of Shavuot with deeper self-knowledge, ready to hear God's word.

Our Passover liberation journey is merely a portal, a gateway to Shavuot.

כַּוָנוֹת הַגּוּף *Kavanot HaGuf*

INTENTIONS FOR THE BODY

Harmonizing with Balance and Dynamic Tension

In our Counting the Omer yoga practice, we explore the dimensions of **Triangle**, **Pyramid**, and **Revolved Triangle Poses**. As we embody these physical configurations, we internalize the spiritual attributes of stability, strength, and discipline alongside freedom, beauty, self-expression, and humility. In **Triangle Pose**, we draw inward with stability and extend outward with strength. Steadying ourselves, we then let go, humbly lowering our heads into **Pyramid Pose**. In the dynamic expression of **Revolved Triangle Pose**, we root, revolve, and beautifully evolve. These postures provide a structure through which to harmonize and balance a wide range of energies and potentials within and around us.

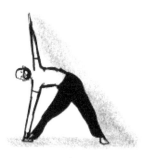
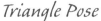
Triangle Pose

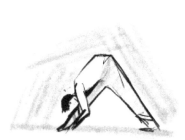
Pyramid Pose

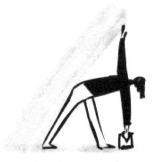
Revolved Triangle Pose

Triangle Pose

- Start with the legs approximately three feet apart. Rotate the right front foot out and pivot the left foot in. Align the heels and ground down with the feet.
- Widen both arms out, shoulder height and parallel to the floor. Extend the right arm long.
- While keeping the legs straight and strong, reach out and down to touch toward the right foot and stretch the left arm up. Maintain awareness of both shoulder blades tracking down the back. Widen the chest and lengthen both sides of the waist.
- Engage the core muscles. Remain in **Triangle Pose** for 5 cycles of breath, feeling the strength and length of the torso. Root down to rise out of the pose, and repeat on the other side.

Pyramid Pose

- Step back with the left foot approximately one leg length. Root and ground the feet. Tone the leg muscles. Allow the feet to be wide enough apart to feel steady and balanced. Orient both feet and hips to face forward.
- Straighten both knees. Tone the navel up and in. Then cascade the upper body over the front leg. Draw the shoulders away from the ears. Feel the humble and introspective nature of lowering the head into **Pyramid Pose**. Maintain the pose for 5 cycles of breath.

Revolved Triangle Pose

- Continue to stabilize the lower body, pressing into the back foot. Place the left hand on the hip. Then move the left hand across the midline to

YOUR YOGA SEQUENCE

לִסְפּוֹר *Lispor* To Count

*Focusing on the Hebrew word above, create and expand upon
your own yoga practice. Embody the themes of the holiday.*

- a space for divine inspiration & practical ideas -

the right foot. Lengthen, extend, and lean the torso back, turning to the
right. Draw the right hip back, stacking the shoulders, extending the
right arm, and gazing up in **Revolved Triangle Pose**.

- For 5 cycles of breath, focus on the right hand, striving to maintain
balance while standing in this beautiful and dynamic expression of a
twist. Enjoy the relationship of body and mind in harmony.

- Release and repeat **Pyramid** to **Revolved Triangle Pose** on the other side.

Find a seat for meditation.
Close the eyes.
With an alert spine, settle into stillness.
Observe the breath.
Notice any sounds. Feel the air on the skin.
Become present.

With eyes closed, rock very slightly on your seat. Come to stillness, a place of balance with awareness equally distributed between the tripod of the sitting bones and the pubic bone. Each bone, each aspect of our lives, each breath, counts. Quietly whisper the word: לִסְפּוֹר, *"Lispor."*

Scan the face, moving the awareness in a triangular pattern from the ears to the mouth and chin. Relax the eye region and move the awareness from the eyes to the very center of the brain.

Feel the weight of the shoulders in relation to the back. Sense the balance and spaciousness around the heart and lungs. Take an accounting of the body, and again whisper the word: לִסְפּוֹר, *"Lispor."*

Now, move the awareness down into the belly. Take a deep breath. Then, witness awareness as it travels into the pelvis, lower back, and legs. Sense the symmetry and balance held in the physical realm. See the body as a sacred vessel, able to hold many emotions, truths, memories, dreams, and realities.

Feel the body, balanced and whole.

Slowly, when ready, open the eyes.

Write or draw.

In what area of my life do I experience balance?

In what area of my life am I lacking balance?

How might I lean in or lean away, intensify, or release
לִסְפּוֹר, *lispor* (to make each moment count)
and establish greater harmony, flow, and fulfillment in my life?

Teach us to number our days, that we may obtain a heart of wisdom.

PSALM 90:12

10
Shavuot

Receiving Torah at Mount Sinai

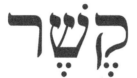

Kesher • Connection

How deeply You have loved us, Adonai,
gracing us with surpassing compassion...
Enlighten us with Torah. Focus our minds on acts of holiness.
Unite our hearts in love and awe for Your name.

FROM THE BLESSING WHICH PRECEDES
THE MORNING RECITATION OF THE SHEMA*

---

* The wording selection of this prayer has been adapted by Tara Feldman, drawn from *Mishkan T'filah: A Reform Siddur* (CCAR Press, 2007).

HOLIDAY TRADITIONS

Embracing Covenant

- Shavuot is one of three annual pilgrimage festivals, celebrated since ancient times by journeying to Jerusalem.

- Shavuot celebrates the receiving of Torah at Mount Sinai.

- The Hebrew word Shavuot means "weeks." This holiday falls at the end of the seven-week Counting of the Omer, which begins on the second day of Passover.

- The holiday commences with an all-night Torah study session, leading into morning prayers during which the Ten Commandments are read.

- Shavuot observance also includes reading from the Book of Ruth which tells the story of Ruth, a non-Jewish Moabite woman who chose to convert and to align her life and her fate with that of the Jewish people.

- It is traditional on Shavuot to eat cheesecake and other foods made with dairy products. Those living in Israel mark the holiday by celebrating the first fruits of the season.

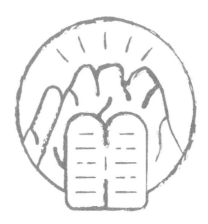

כַּוָּנוֹת הַנֶּפֶשׁ *Kavanot HaNefesh*

INTENTIONS FOR THE SOUL

Heaven Touches Earth

Shavuot invokes themes of love, interconnection, and awe. Receiving Torah in the wilderness of Sinai sealed the covenant between God and the Jewish people. It is taught that all Jewish souls who were yet to come into the world were present at the moment of revelation when God's truth pierced human consciousness. The ancient rabbinic imagination describes this mystical event in vastly different ways. Perhaps it was an experience of cacophonous sound, of thunder and lightning. Perhaps it was an experience of sublime silence. Whatever actually occurred at Mount Sinai, this experience left the Jewish people changed forever, bound to God.

All Jewish souls who were yet to come into the world were present at that moment when God's truth pierced human consciousness.

כַּוָּנוֹת הַגּוּף *Kavanot HaGuf*

INTENTIONS FOR THE BODY

Entwining, Embracing, and Binding in Commitment and Love

In our Shavuot yoga practice, we stimulate the life-force energy through postures that bind, entwine, and wrap the limbs around the central axis of the body. The essential postures of **Eagle Pose** and **Seated Twist Pose** awaken an inner spark. We draw in, compress, and then release our limbs from the midline, emerging, ecstatic, reenergized and recharged. Our spirits soaring, we affirm the eternal contract bestowed upon us—a commitment to ourselves, to community, and to God.

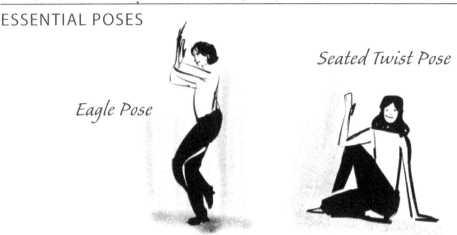

Eagle Pose

Seated Twist Pose

Eagle Pose

- Stand with both feet on the ground, bend the knees slightly, and shift the weight to the right foot. Lift the left leg. Wrap and entwine the left leg over the right leg, balancing on the right foot. Squeeze the inner thighs together, and tuck the toes behind the calf.
- Bend both elbows at a 90-degree angle, and slip the left upper arm under the right arm. Narrow and hug the forearms around each other. Hook the wrists, and join the palms together with thumbs resting between the eyebrows at the "third eye."
- Draw the limbs inward toward the midline. Here, in **Eagle Pose**, feel the spark. Embrace the union of opposites. Breathe for 5 cycles.
- Unwind, recover, and repeat on the other side.

Seated Twist Pose

- Come to a seat. Bend both knees, and place the soles of the feet on the ground. Cross the right foot over to the outside of the left thigh, firmly planting the sole into the earth.
- Inhaling, sit up tall, and reach the left arm up toward the sky, elongating the spine. As you exhale, turn to the right, pressing the bent left elbow against the outer right thigh. Place the left arm at the outer right knee to open the chest. Gaze over the right shoulder. Remain in this **Seated Twist Pose** for 5 cycles of breath.
- Optionally, to deepen and challenge the twist, slide the left arm under the right leg and wrap the right hand behind the back to clasp and bind with the left hand.
- Feel the *kesher* (connection). Then, unwind, and release the pose. Repeat on the other side.

קֶשֶׁר *Kesher* Connection

Focusing on the Hebrew word above, create and expand upon your own yoga practice. Embody the themes of the holiday.

- a space for divine inspiration & practical ideas -

GUIDED MEDITATION

Find a seat for meditation.
Close the eyes.
With an alert spine, settle into stillness.
Observe the breath.
Notice any sounds. Feel the air on the skin.
Become present.

Feel the body grounded and erect, solid and majestic as a mountain. Allow the shoulders to drop, and with each breath, sense energy ascending and descending along the spinal column and central axis of the body. Bring awareness to the heart center. Become still enough to sense the beating heart.

Invite into consciousness the invisible, mysterious channels of connection which organize and bind self, community, and loved ones. Honor those connections. Quietly whisper the word: קֶשֶׁר, *"Kesher."*

Now, envision being surrounded by light, a protective radiance, starting at the crown of the head and descending down throughout the body. Imagine a Divine, protective Presence infusing the body and saturating each breath. Again, whisper the word: קֶשֶׁר, *"Kesher."*

Slowly, when ready, open the eyes.

JOURNALING

Write or draw.

In what area of my life do I experience or have I experienced קֶשֶׁר, *kesher* (a deep sense of connection)?

Where do I seek deeper connection?

What do I want to learn in the coming months?
How can I make my learning an act of love?

If a love depends on a something, when that thing ceases, the love ceases; but a love that does not depend on anything, will never cease.

PIRKE AVOT, THE ETHICS OF THE FATHERS 5:16

11
Tisha B'Av

Commemorating the Destruction of the Temple

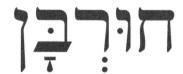

Hurban · Destruction

When we are no longer able to change a situation,
we are challenged to change ourselves.

VIKTOR FRANKL

HOLIDAY TRADITIONS

Mourning, Remembrance and Loss

- Tisha B'Av, the ninth day of the Hebrew month Av, commemorates the destruction of the First and Second Temples in Jerusalem in the years 586 BCE and 70 CE.

- The holiday is a day of mourning, which includes reading from *Eicha* (the Book of Lamentations), the recitation of *kinot* (mournful prayers), observing a 25-hour fast, and refraining from washing and acts of physical pleasure or luxury.

- Tisha B'Av is preceded by three weeks of solemnity in which traditional communities abstain from celebration—and on Shabbat, prophetic readings of warning and rebuke are offered.

- During the final nine days leading up to Tisha B'Av, the atmosphere of mourning is intensified.

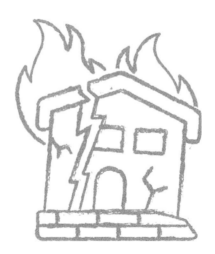

כַּוָּנוֹת הַנֶּפֶשׁ *Kavanot HaNefesh*

INTENTIONS FOR THE SOUL

Destruction and Rebirth

Tisha B'Av has come to memorialize not only the Jewish expulsion from ancient Israel but the persecution of Jews throughout the ages—and even the brokenness of our world at large. Themes invoked by the Ninth of Av include vulnerability, desolation, and exile. Fear, grief, and anger are central emotions in the catharsis that defines this holiday. When the Temple in Jerusalem was destroyed, Judaism was compelled to evolve beyond a religion based on priesthood and sacrifices. In fact, it was precisely because of the destruction of Jerusalem that rabbinic Judaism emerged with study of Torah, prayer, and righteous deeds as the new foundation of Jewish life. Thus, even as Tisha B'Av focuses on destruction, the tragedies which this holiday commemorates create a space for rebirth.

When the Temple in Jerusalem was destroyed,
Jewish life was compelled to evolve.

כַּוָּנוֹת הַגּוּף *Kavanot HaGuf*

INTENTIONS FOR THE BODY

Facing Destruction in Brokenness and Exile

For Tisha B'Av, our Yin Yoga practice moves toward introspection. As opposed to the more energetic, muscular Yang Yoga style, Yin Yoga gives us the structure to settle into passivity, darkness, coolness, stillness, and to the slow passage of time. The practice of Yin Yoga is rooted in ancient Chinese Yin Yang philosophy, traditional Chinese medicine (TCM), and organ-meridian theory. Our practice includes low-to-the-ground poses, such as **Swan**, **Sphinx**, **Reclining Twist**, and **Corpse Poses**. These poses stimulate the subtle energy channels as well as the connective and soft tissues of the body. With an observer's mind, we uncover buried edges of sensation and emotion. Yin Yoga provides an entryway into the realm of the mysterious, the dark, and the hidden. This practice, especially on Tisha B'Av, can be a catalyst to recognize our inherited despair caused by exile, anti-Semitism, and other experiences of trauma and loss. We emerge from a Yin Yoga practice with heightened sensitivity, deepened understanding, and expanded subtle awareness.

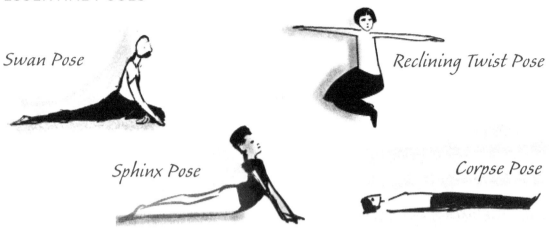

Swan Pose

Reclining Twist Pose

Sphinx Pose

Corpse Pose

Swan Pose

- Come onto the floor on the hands and knees. Slide the right knee forward and the left leg back. Use any props such as a blanket or pillow so that the hips remain even and still.
- Release the ribs, shoulders, and head toward the floor. Bending over the front leg, come to stillness in **Swan Pose**.
- Maintain the pose for approximately 5 minutes, observing any sensations, feelings, or thoughts that arise.
- To recover, move with more active yang energy into a counterpose such as **Downward Facing Dog Pose** (see page 100 in the Yoga Appendix). Repeat **Swan Pose** on the other side.

Sphinx Pose

- Begin prone, face down. Prop up onto the forearms with the elbows bent. Lift the chest up into **Sphinx Pose**. The head can remain upright, or the neck can be relaxed and the head lowered.
- Optionally, extend the elbows and straighten the arms to deepen the sensation. Remain in this pose for 5 minutes.
- Recovering from the pose, slowly lower to the ground from the backbend and remain on the belly. Make windshield wiper motions with the lower legs to release and reenergize the lower back.

Reclining Twist Pose

- Turn onto the back in a supine position, bending both knees. Open the arms wide at shoulder height and draw the shoulder blades down the back. Drop the knees to the right, stacking one knee on top of the other.

חוּרְבָּן *Hurban* Destruction

*Focusing on the Hebrew word above, create and expand upon
your own yoga practice. Embody the themes of the holiday.*

- a space for divine inspiration & practical ideas -

- Lengthen the tailbone away from the chest. Turn the neck and head to the left. Remain in **Reclining Twist Pose** for 5 minutes.
- Repeat on the other side.

Corpse Pose

- Lie on the back in **Corpse Pose**, releasing the body to the floor. Allow the limbs to drop away from the midline of the body. Turn the palms to face up and the feet to splay out.
- Draw the shoulder blades together to facilitate heart opening and to release tension from the body.
- Close the eyes. Let the breath become easy and natural, emptying the mind. Remain in this pose for at least 5 minutes. Acknowledge *hurban* (destruction), and let go.

מֶדִיטַצְיָה מוּדְרֶכֶת *Meditatziyah Mudrechet*

GUIDED MEDITATION

Find a seat for meditation.
Close the eyes.
With an alert spine, settle into stillness.
Observe the breath.
Notice any sounds. Feel the air on the skin.
Become present.

Recall a moment of destruction. Encounter the experience of loss. Breathe fully. As you exhale, whisper the word: חוּרְבָּן, *"Hurban."*

Now, rest the hands on the thighs with palms turned down. Experience the sorrow of that which is no more. Create space to feel the reality of loss, to know grief. Again, whisper the word: חוּרְבָּן, *"Hurban."*

Now, place the hands on the sternum one on top of the other. Feel the beating heart. Acknowledge the presence of self and of God.

Return the hands to the thighs with palms turned upward. Relax any tension in the shoulders, neck, and face. Breathe in healing. Breathe out compassion. With a cleansing breath, open to faith and trust, to resilience and transformation—a journey that continues.

Slowly, when ready, open the eyes.

JOURNALING

Write or draw.

In what area of my life do I experience or have I experienced חוּרְבָּן, *hurban* (loss and destruction)?

What loss has been among the hardest?

How has this loss changed me, and how might I use it to evolve toward my future with hope?

Alas! Lonely sits the city once great with people!
Bitterly she weeps in the night, her cheek wet with tears.
Of all her friends, there is none to comfort her.
All her allies have betrayed her. They have become her foes.

LAMENTATIONS 1: 1-2

12

Elul

Preparing the Soul
to Begin Again

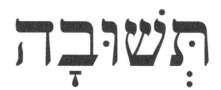

Teshuvah • Return

The gates of prayer are sometimes open and sometimes closed,
but the gates of teshuvah are always open.

MIDRASH, DEVARIM RABBAH 2:12

HOLIDAY TRADITIONS

Reflection, Return and Renewal

- The month of Elul concludes the annual cycle of the Jewish calendar and leads into Rosh HaShanah.

- Throughout the 29 days of Elul, we request forgiveness from those we may have hurt and open our hearts to the possibility of forgiveness.

- Every weekday morning during this month, the *shofar* (ram's horn) is sounded.

- Other Elul practices include reciting Psalm 27, offering *selichot* (penitential prayers), and visiting the graves of loved ones.

- The Hebrew letters which spell the word Elul form an acronym (in Hebrew) for verse 6:3 from the Song of Songs, "I am my beloved's and my beloved is mine."

- During Elul, Jews reaffirm the bonds between themselves and loved ones, their connection to community, and the eternal covenant between God and the Jewish people.

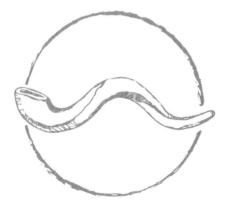

כַּוָּנוֹת הַנֶּפֶשׁ *Kavanot HaNefesh*

INTENTIONS FOR THE SOUL

Preparing the Soul to Begin Again

Elul awakens in us the hope for renewal. It is a month of personal reflection, which prepares us to enter the New Year as our best selves. As with the entire High Holy Days season, the journey of Elul is enacted through: 1. *tefillah*—prayer (inner self-examination and communion with God); 2. *teshuvah*—repentance (returning to our better selves); and 3. *tzedakah*—charity (giving monetary resources to promote the values of *tzedek*—justice, and *hesed*—compassion). Elul is a time of honest self-assessment, a month to recommit ourselves to that which matters most. As summer turns to fall, we acknowledge the passage of time and the reality that each of us is mortal. Inspired by this awareness, we pray to be inscribed in the Book of Life for a year of meaning and blessing.

Elul is a time of honest self-assessment, a month to recommit ourselves to that which matters most.

כַּוָּנוֹת הַגּוּף *Kavanot HaGuf*

INTENTIONS FOR THE BODY

Assessing the Past, Preparing for the Future

Our Elul yoga practice encompasses the past, present, and future. We acknowledge the year gone by. We ground ourselves in the present. Finally, we open our hearts and minds to the future. Our practice offers three essential postures:

- Past/*Tefillah*—**Standing Forward Bend Pose**: Forward bends are calming for the mind and the nervous system. They orient our gaze inward, facilitating introspection.

- Present/*Teshuvah*—**Revolved Low Lunge Pose**: Twists stimulate and mobilize stagnant energy. They bring on the capacity for change, renewal, and transformation.

- Future/*Tzedakah*—**Dancer pose**: In yoga, backbends are affectionately referred to as "heart openers." They generate energy and expand blood flow, reminding us to be vital, courageous, and compassionate in our pursuit of righteous action.

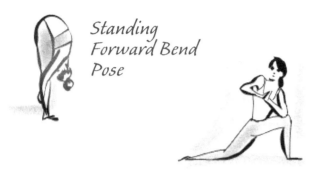

Standing Forward Bend Pose

Revolved Low Lunge Pose

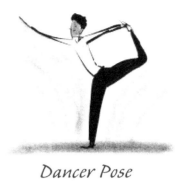

Dancer Pose

Standing Forward Bend Pose

- From a standing position, align the hips over the heels. Elongate the spine. Lift the navel, and then hinge into a forward fold over the legs. Work to straighten the legs. Draw the shoulders away from the ears.
- With the head released down and the focus turned inward, observe yourself in **Standing Forward Bend Pose**. Breathe for 5 cycles as you reflect upon and consider the past year.

Revolved Low Lunge Pose

- From the **Standing Forward Bend**, step the left leg back. Lowering the left knee to the floor, come into a low lunge. Press the shoulders away from the ears. Inhale the hands together at the heart center, lifting the torso. Exhale and rotate the left elbow to the outside of the right (front) thigh.
- Spin the chest open. Sense the stimulating energy that **Revolved Low Lunge Pose** can bring to the central axis of the body, including the musculoskeletal, digestive, and nervous systems. For a variation, lift the left (back) knee off the ground.
- As you breathe for 5 cycles in this pose, imagine a change that you would like to manifest this year, a challenge you would like to move through.
- Unwind, and return to a standing position. Repeat the **Revolved Low Lunge** sequence on the other side.

Dancer Pose

- Begin standing with both feet on the ground. Shift the weight to the right foot, and bend the left knee back. Reach behind with the left hand to hold

תְּשׁוּבָה *Teshuvah* Return

*Focusing on the Hebrew word above, create and expand upon
your own yoga practice. Embody the themes of the holiday.*

- a space for divine inspiration & practical ideas -

---

the outside of the left foot. Keep the standing leg straight. Lift the thigh
upward in **Dancer Pose**.

- Expand at the chest, opening around the heart. Reach the opposite arm
forward, with the palm of the hand facing upward.
- Play with the balance, envisioning the future ahead. Breathe for 5 cycles.
- Release, and repeat the sequence on the other side.

GUIDED MEDITATION

Find a seat for meditation.
Close the eyes.
With an alert spine, settle into stillness.
Observe the breath.
Notice any sounds. Feel the air on the skin.
Become present.

With the mind's eye, consider the flow of time. Review the year that has passed. Allow memories, impressions, events and moments to arise. Think back to last fall, winter, spring, summer. What is the "harvest" of this season? Feel the fullness of the past year.

Now, let the mind and heart settle on one moment of fulfillment from the year gone by. Linger here, allowing for gratitude. Remain conscious of the breath.

With another cycle of breath, come into the present moment. Consider an ongoing personal challenge. In facing this challenge, what questions arise? Whisper the word: תְּשׁוּבָה, *"Teshuvah."*

Imagine stepping toward and into this challenge with hope and trust. Envision making one small choice which symbolizes change, transformation. Whisper the word: תְּשׁוּבָה, *"Teshuvah."*

Slowly, when ready, open the eyes.

Write or draw.

What is the harvest of the year gone by?

What is a challenge that I currently face?

How can I use this challenge to make תְּשׁוּבָה, *teshuvah,* and offer צְדָקָה, *tzedakah,* to rise up, transform and grow?

One thing I ask of the God. Only this do I seek:
to live in God's house all the days of my life,
to gaze upon God's beauty, to frequent God's temple.

PSALM 27:4

YOGA PRACTICE TEMPLATE

Holiday: Essential Poses:

Mantra: Chants/Prayers/Readings:

Warm-Up Sequence:

Hip Openers:

Twists / Core Work: Inversions:

Backbends:

Forward Bends: Cool-Down Poses:

Yoga Appendix

Sun Salutations

Sun Salutations are to be practiced in sequence, coordinating movement with breath.

Mountain Pose	Extended Mountain Pose	Forward Bend Pose	Lunge Pose

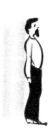 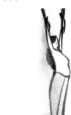 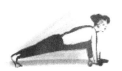

Downward Facing Dog Pose	Plank Pose	Pushup Pose	Cobra Pose/ Sphinx Pose

  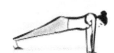 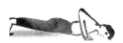 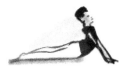

Downward Facing Dog Pose	Lunge Pose	Forward Bend Pose

 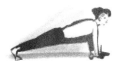

Extended Mountain Pose	Mountain Pose

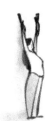 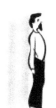

Warm-up Poses and Sequences

Begin each session with Warm-up Poses and Sequences, which create focus and heat, so the practice of yoga can proceed with clarity and safety. Listen, assess, and connect to the alignment and intentions of the body, breath, and spirit.

Easy Seat Pose   Cat and Cow Poses   Child's Pose

 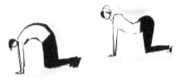 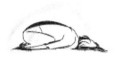

Grounding Poses

Grounding Poses stabilize and strengthen the body. By rooting through the feet and firming the legs, these poses establish energetic presence and confidence.

Hero Pose   Chair Pose   Downward Facing Dog Pose

  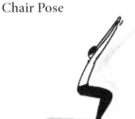 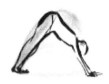

Warrior I Pose   Warrior II Pose

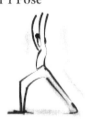 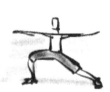

Hip Opening Poses

Hip Opening Poses facilitate flexibility and stability around the hip joints, legs, and buttocks. These poses encourage blood flow: softening tension where there is restriction; increasing range of motion and freedom where there is limitation.

Lunge Pose   Straddle Pose   Garland Pose

 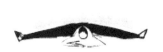

Full Split Pose   Full Split Pose Variation   Pigeon Pose/Swan Pose

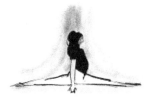 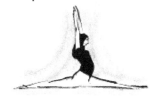 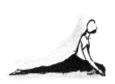

Side Bending Poses

Side Bending Poses promote symmetry in the spine and awareness of the torso. These poses create space for the lungs to expand and the capacity to breathe more deeply. In addition, side bends allow for movement beyond the expected confines of the self, opening and energizing the practitioner toward new horizons.

Side Angle Pose   Gate Pose   Triangle Pose   Peaceful Warrior Pose

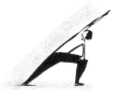

Core Strengthening Poses

Core Strengthening Poses awaken, strengthen, and tone the torso with an emphasis on the abdominal muscles. These poses stimulate and energize the body and mind, burning off stagnation and lethargy.

Plank Pose   Table Top Pose   Boat Pose   Forearm Plank Pose

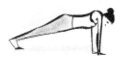 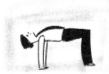 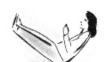 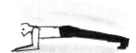

Standing Balance Poses

Standing Balance Poses tone the muscles, bones, and ligaments of the feet and legs. These poses promote physical and energetic balance and alignment, encouraging fortitude, stability, and concentration.

Tree pose   Eagle Pose   Dancer Pose   Warrior III Pose

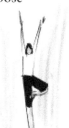 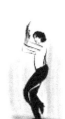 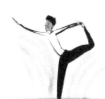 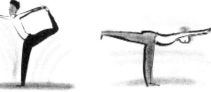

Inversion Poses

Inversion Poses are physically and mentally stimulating. Inversions challenge, strengthen, and invigorate the body, requiring keen concentration and steady presence. As the head is aligned below the heart and the blood flow to the organs of the body is reversed, these poses have the potential to elicit healing and transformation.

Downward Facing Dog Pose

Headstand Pose

Shoulderstand Pose

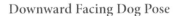
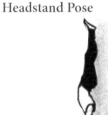

Plough Pose

Forward Bend Pose

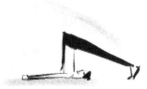
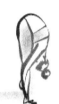

Twisting Poses

Twisting Poses tone and stimulate the abdomen, stretch the back and chest muscles, and relieve tension in the spine. Twisting poses mobilize physical and emotional energy and have the capacity to alleviate feelings of being "blocked" or "stuck."

Seated Twist Pose

Seated Twist Pose Variation

Revolved Triangle Pose

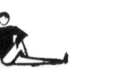

Revolved Low Lunge Pose

Revolved Chair Pose

Reclining Twist Pose

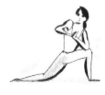

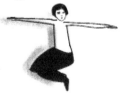

Back Bending Poses

Back Bending Poses extend and strengthen the back of the body, opening and stretching the front of the body. Affectionately referred to as "heart openers," backbends stimulate vitality and challenge the practitioner to expand with heartfelt vigor.

Sphinx Pose   Locust Pose   Camel Pose

Bow Pose   Wheel Pose   Fish Pose   Bridge Pose

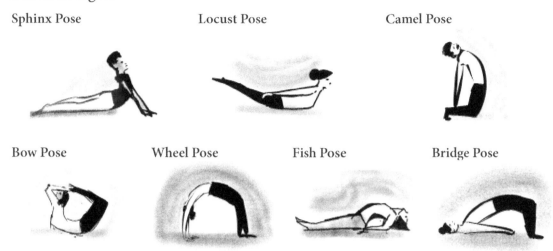

Forward Bending and Closing Poses

Forward Bending and Closing Poses lengthen and relax the body. They release tension and are calming. With eyes relaxed and the gaze turned inward, these poses cool the nervous system and facilitate introspection. Promoting inner harmony and peace, these poses provide an entryway for meditation and prayer.

Puppy Dog Pose   Child's Pose   Full Pranam Pose

Forward Bend Pose   Pyramid Pose   Knees to Chest Pose

Corpse Pose

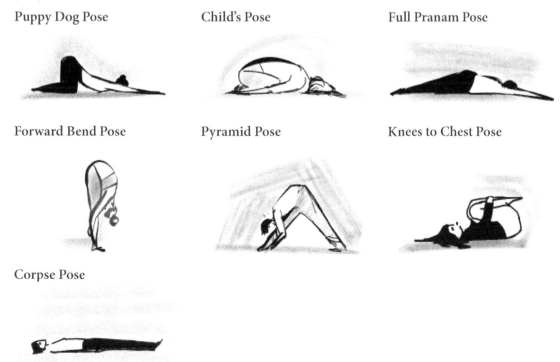

Holiday Chants, Prayers, Songs, and Texts

ROSH HASHANAH

Chant

תְּקַע בְּשׁוֹפָר גָּדוֹל לְחֵרוּתֵנוּ וְשָׂא נֵס לְקַבֵּץ גָּלִיּוֹתֵינוּ

T'kah b'shofar gadol l'cheiruteinu. V'sa neis l'kabeitz galuyoteinu.

Sound the great shofar for our freedom,
and raise the banner as we all come home.[1]

Prayers

Blessings for eating apples dipped in honey

בָּרוּךְ אַתָּה יְיָ אֱלֹהֵינוּ מֶלֶךְ הָעוֹלָם. בּוֹרֵא פְּרִי הָעֵץ

Baruch atah Adonai, Eloheinu melech ha'olam, borei p'ri ha'eitz.

Blessed are You, Adonai, our God, Sovereign of the Universe, Creator of the
fruit of the tree.

יְהִי רָצוֹן מִלְפָנֶךָ יְיָ אֱלֹהֵינוּ וֵאלֹהֵי אֲבוֹתֵינוּ וְאִמוֹתֵינוּ
שֶׁתְּחַדֵּשׁ עָלֵינוּ שָׁנָה טוֹבָה וּמְתוּקָה

*Y'hi ratzon milfanechah, Adonai Eloheinu v'Elohei avoteinu v'imoteinu
shetchadeish aleinu shanah tovah um'tukah.*

May it be Your will, Adonai our God and God of our fathers and mothers,
that we be renewed for a good and sweet new year.

Blessings for hearing the shofar

בָּרוּךְ אַתָּה יְהֹוָה אֱלֹהֵינוּ מֶלֶךְ הָעוֹלָם אֲשֶׁר קִדְּשָׁנוּ בְּמִצְוֹתָיו וְצִוָּנוּ לִשְׁמֹעַ קוֹל שׁוֹפָר

*Baruch atah Adonai, Eloheinu melech ha'olam, asher kidshanu b'mitzvotav
v'tzivanu lishmo'ah kol shofar.*

Blessed are You, Adonai, our God, Sovereign of the Universe, Who sanctifies
us with mitzvot and commands us to hear the call of the shofar.

---

1. *Freedom and Homecoming: T'ka B'Shofar,* https://www.rabbishefagold.com/freedom-homecoming/
2. Translations of all prayers and blessings in this book are adapted from *Mishkan T'filah, A Reform
   Siddur* (CCAR Press, 2007).

Holiday Song

לְשָׁנָה טוֹבָה תִּכָּתֵבוּ וְתֵחָתֵמוּ

L'Shanah tovah tikateivu v'teichateimu.

May you be inscribed and sealed for a good year.

YOM KIPPUR

Chant

קַח נָא אֶת נַפְשִׁי מִמֶּנִּי

Kach nah et nafshi mimeni.

Take my life.

—Jonah 4:3 [3]

Prayers

Ashamnu/Viddui—Confession of Sin [4]

אָשַׁמְנוּ—*Ashamnu.* We betray.

בָּגַדְנוּ—*Bagadnu.* We steal.

גָּזַלְנוּ—*Gazalnu.* We scorn.

דִּבַּרְנוּ דֹפִי—*Dibarnu dofi.* We act perversely.

הֶעֱוִינוּ—*He'evinu.* We are cruel.

וְהִרְשַׁעְנוּ—*V'hirshanu.* We scheme.

זַדְנוּ—*Zadnu.* We sin with bad intent.

חָמַסְנוּ—*Chamasnu.* We are violent.

טָפַלְנוּ שֶׁקֶר—*Tafalnu shaker.* We slander.

יָעַצְנוּ רָע—*Ya'atznu rah.* We devise evil.

לַצְנוּ—*Latznu.* We lie.

כִּזַּבְנוּ—*Kizavnu.* We ridicule.

מָרַדְנוּ—*Maradnu.* We disobey.

נִאַצְנוּ—*Ni'atznu.* We abuse.

סָרַרְנוּ—*Sararnu.* We defy.

עָוִינוּ—*Avinu.* We corrupt.

פָּשַׁעְנוּ—*Pashanu.* We commit crimes.

צָרַרְנוּ—*Tzararnu.* We are hostile.

קִשִּׁינוּ עֹרֶף—*Kishinu oref.* We are stiff-necked.

---

3. *Surrendering the Small Self: Kach Nah,* https://www.rabbishefagold.com/surrendering-small-self/

4. Translation based on and adapted from *The Metsudah Machzor* (via Sefaria.org) and *Mishkan Hanefesh: Machzor for the Days of Awe: Yom Kippur* (CCAR Press, 2015).

רָשַׁעְנוּ—*Rashanu.* We are immoral.

שִׁחַתְנוּ—*Shichatnu.* We kill.

תִּעַבְנוּ—*Ti'avnu.* We spoil.

תָּעִינוּ—*Ta'inu.* We go astray.

תִּעְתָּעְנוּ—*Titanu.* We lead others astray.

Avinu Malkeinu

אָבִינוּ מַלְכֵּנוּ חָנֵּנוּ וַעֲנֵנוּ כִּי אֵין בָּנוּ מַעֲשִׂים עֲשֵׂה עִמָּנוּ צְדָקָה וָחֶסֶד וְהוֹשִׁיעֵנוּ

Avinu Malkeinu, chaneinu va'aneinu ki ein banu ma'asim.
Asei imanu tzedakah va'hesed v'hoshi'einu.

Our Father, our King, be gracious to us and answer us for we have little merit.
Treat us with righteousness and kindness and deliver us.

SUKKOT

Chant

אֶת הַכֹּל עָשָׂה יָפֶה בְעִתּוֹ גַּם אֶת־הָעֹלָם נָתַן בְּלִבָּם

Et hakol asah yafeh b'ito, gam et ha'olam natan b'libam.

God makes everything beautiful in its time,
and also hides the universe in their hearts.
—Ecclesiastes 3:11 [5]

Prayers

Blessing for dwelling in the sukkah

בָּרוּךְ אַתָּה יְהֹוָה אֱלֹהֵינוּ מֶלֶךְ הָעוֹלָם אֲשֶׁר קִדְּשָׁנוּ בְּמִצְוֹתָיו וְצִוָּנוּ לֵישֵׁב בַּסֻּכָּה

Baruch atah Adonai Eloheinu melech ha'olam, asher kidshanu bamitzvotav,
v'tzivanu leisheiv ba'sukkah.

Blessed are You, Adonai our God, Sovereign of the Universe, Who sanctifies us
with mitzvot and has commanded us to sit in the sukkah.

Blessing for shaking the lulav

בָּרוּךְ אַתָּה יְהֹוָה אֱלֹהֵינוּ מֶלֶךְ הָעוֹלָם. אֲשֶׁר קִדְּשָׁנוּ בְּמִצְוֹתָיו וְצִוָּנוּ עַל נְטִילַת לוּלָב

Baruch atah Adonai, Eloheinu melech ha'olam, asher kidshanu bamitzvotav,
v'tzivanu al n'tilat lulav.

Blessed are You, Adonai our God, Sovereign of the Universe, Who sanctifies us
with mitzvot and has commanded us to raise up the lulav.

---

5. *Knowing Beauty and Finding the Universe: Et Kol Asa,* https://www.rabbishefagold.com/
knowing-beauty-universe/

Biblical Text

לְכֹל זְמָן וְעֵת לְכָל־חֵפֶץ תַּחַת הַשָּׁמָיִם

Lakol z'man, v'eit l'chol heifetz tachat hashamayim.

A season is set for everything, a time for every experience under heaven:

A time to be born and a time to die,

A time to plant and a time to uproot the planted,

A time to slay and a time to heal,

A time to tear down and a time to build up,

A time to weep and a time to laugh,

A time for wailing and a time for dancing,

A time to throw stones and a time to gather stones,

A time to embrace and a time to refrain from embracing,

A time to seek and a time to lose,

A time to keep and a time to discard,

A time to tear and a time to sew,

A time to keep silence and a time to speak,

A time to love and a time to hate,

A time for war and a time for peace.

—Ecclesiastes 3:1-8 [6]

SIMCHAT TORAH

Chant

Hilulah, hilulah, hilulah, Halleluyah!

כֹּל הַנְּשָׁמָה תְּהַלֵּל יָהּ הַלְלוּ יָהּ

Kol han'shamah t'haleilyah.

Let all that breathes praise God. Halleluyah.

—Psalm 150:6 [7]

Prayers

Blessings for before and after Torah reading

בָּרְכוּ אֶת יְיָ הַמְבֹרָךְ

Barchu et Adonai ham'vorach.

Bless Adonai Who is blessed.

---

6. Text and translation of all Biblical passages in this book are adapted from sefaria.org.

7. *Celebration in Praise: Kol Ha'n'shama,* https://www.rabbishefagold.com/praise/

בָּרוּךְ יְיָ הַמְבֹרָךְ לְעוֹלָם וָעֶד

Baruch Adonai ham'vorach l'olam va'ed.

Blessed is Adonai Who is blessed forever.

בָּרוּךְ אַתָּה יְיָ אֱלֹהֵינוּ מֶלֶךְ הָעוֹלָם אֲשֶׁר בָּחַר בָּנוּ מִכָּל הָעַמִּים
וְנָתַן לָנוּ אֶת תּוֹרָתוֹ. בָּרוּךְ אַתָּה יְיָ נוֹתֵן הַתּוֹרָה

*Baruch atah Adonai, eloheinu melech ha'olam, asher bachar banu mikol
ha'amim, v'natan lanu et torato. Baruch atah Adonai, notein haTorah.*

Blessed are You, Adonai, our God, Sovereign of the Universe, Who has chosen
us from among the peoples and given us the Torah. Blessed are You, God,
Who gives the Torah.

בָּרוּךְ אַתָּה יְיָ אֱלֹהֵינוּ מֶלֶךְ הָעוֹלָם אֲשֶׁר נָתַן לָנוּ תּוֹרַת אֱמֶת
וְחַיֵּי עוֹלָם נָטַע בְּתוֹכֵנוּ. בָּרוּךְ אַתָּה יְיָ נוֹתֵן הַתּוֹרָה

*Baruch atah Adonai, eloheinu melech ha'olam, asher natan lanu Torat emet,
v'chayei olam natah b'tocheinu. Baruch atah Adonai notein haTorah.*

Blessed are You, Adonai, our God, Sovereign of the Universe,
Who has given us a Torah of truth, implanting within us eternal life.
Blessed are You, God, Who gives the Torah.

Prayer offered during hakafot [8]

לְמַעַנְךָ אֱלֹהֵינוּ הוֹשַׁע נָא: לְמַעַנְךָ בּוֹרְאֵנוּ הוֹשַׁע נָא

L'ma'anchah Eloheinu hoshiya nah. L'ma'anchah Boreinu hoshiah nah.

For Your sake, our God, save us. For Your sake, our Creator, save us!

HANUKKAH

Chant

אֵשׁ תָּמִיד תּוּקַד עַל־הַמִּזְבֵּחַ לֹא תִכְבֶּה

Aish tamid tukad al hamizbei'ach lo tichbeh.

Fire always shall be kept burning on the altar. It shall not go out.
—Leviticus 6:6 [9]

---

8. The term *hakafah*, and the plural *hakafot*, refer to circular processions while holding a Torah scroll.
9. *Fire on the Altar: Aish Tamid,* https://www.rabbishefagold.com/fire-on-altar-aish-tamid/

Prayers

Blessing for kindling the Hanukkah lights

FIRST BLESSING

בָּרוּךְ אַתָּה יְיָ אֱלֹהֵינוּ מֶלֶךְ הָעוֹלָם אֲשֶׁר קִדְּשָׁנוּ בְּמִצְוֹתָיו וְצִוָּנוּ לְהַדְלִיק נֵר חֲנֻכָּה

Baruch atah Adonai Eloheinu melech ha'olam asher kideshanu b'mitzvotav v'tzivanu l'hadlik neir Hanukkah.

Blessed are You, Adonai our God, Sovereign of the Universe, Who sanctifies us with mitzvot and has commanded us to and commanded us to kindle the Hanukkah light.

SECOND BLESSING

בָּרוּךְ אַתָּה יְיָ אֱלֹהֵינוּ מֶלֶךְ הָעוֹלָם שֶׁעָשָׂה נִסִּים לַאֲבוֹתֵינוּ בַּיָּמִים הָהֵם בַּזְּמַן הַזֶּה

Baruch atah Adonai Eloheinu melech ha'olam she'asah nisim la'avoteinu bayamim haheim bazman hazeh.

Blessed are You, Adonai our God, Sovereign of the Universe, Who performed miracles for our foreparents in those days, at this time.

THIRD BLESSING (RECITED ON THE FIRST NIGHT)

בָּרוּךְ אַתָּה יְיָ אֱלֹהֵינוּ מֶלֶךְ הָעוֹלָם שֶׁהֶחֱיָנוּ וְקִיְּמָנוּ וְהִגִּיעָנוּ לַזְּמַן הַזֶּה

Baruch atah Adonai Eloheinu melech ha'olam shehecheyanu v'kiyimanu v'higiyanu laz'man hazeh.

Blessed are You, Adonai our God, Sovereign of the Universe, Who has granted us life, sustained us, and enabled us to reach this season.

Song

Ma'oz Tzur / Rock of Ages

מָעוֹז צוּר יְשׁוּעָתִי לְךָ נָאֶה לְשַׁבֵּחַ
תִּכּוֹן בֵּית תְּפִלָּתִי וְשָׁם תּוֹדָה נְזַבֵּחַ
לְעֵת תָּכִין מַטְבֵּחַ מִצָּר הַמְנַבֵּחַ
אָז אֶגְמוֹר בְּשִׁיר מִזְמוֹר חֲנֻכַּת הַמִּזְבֵּחַ

Ma'oz Tzur yeshu'ati, l'chah na'eh l'shabei'ach.
Tikon beit tefilati, v'sham todah n'zabei'ach.
L'eit tachin matbei'ach mitzar hamnabei'ach
Az egmor b'shir mizmor chanukat ha mizbei'ach.

Rock of Ages let our song Praise Thy saving power;
Thou amidst the raging foes, Wast our sheltering tower.
Furiously they assailed us, But Thine arm availed us,
And Thy word broke their sword, When our own strength failed us.

Chant

כִּי בְשִׂמְחָה תֵצֵאוּ וּבְשָׁלוֹם תּוּבָלוּן
הֶהָרִים וְהַגְּבָעוֹת יִפְצְחוּ לִפְנֵיכֶם רִנָּה וְכָל־עֲצֵי הַשָּׂדֶה יִמְחֲאוּ כָף

Ki v'simchah teitzei'u, u'v'shalom tuvalun.
Heharim v'hagva'ot yif'tz'chu lifneichem rina v'chol atzei hasadeh yimcha'u chaf.
For in joy you will go out, in peace be led across the land; mountains and hills
will burst into song. and the trees of the field will clap their hands.
—Isaiah 55:12 [10]

Prayers

Blessing for eating the fruit of a tree:

בָּרוּךְ אַתָּה יְיָ אֱלֹהֵינוּ מֶלֶךְ הָעוֹלָם בּוֹרֵא פְּרִי הָעֵץ

Baruch atah Adonai, Elo-heinu melech ha'olam, borei pri ha'eitz.
Blessed are You, Adonai our God, Sovereign of the universe,
Who creates the fruit of the tree.

Prayer for connection with nature, self, and God:
Master of the Universe. Grant me the ability to be alone. May it be my custom
to go outdoors each day among the trees and grass, among all growing things.
There may I be alone and enter into prayer, to talk with the One to whom I
belong. May I express there everything in my heart, and may all the foliage of
the field, all the grasses, trees, and plants awake at my coming, to send the pow-
ers of their life into the words of my prayer so that my prayer and speech are
made whole through the life and spirit of all growing things, which are made as
one by their transcendent Source. May I then pour out the words of my heart
before your Presence like water, O God, and lift up my hands to You in worship.
—Rebbe Nachman of Breslov

Holiday Song

אֶרֶץ זָבַת חָלָב וּדְבָשׁ

Eretz zavat chalav ud'vash.
A land flowing with milk and honey.
—Deuteronomy 26:9

---

10. *For in Joy: Ki V'Simcha,* https://www.rabbishefagold.com/for-in-joy-ki-vsimcha/

PURIM

Chant

לֹא נֵדַע מַה נַּעֲבֹד אֶת יְהֹוָה עַד בֹּאֵנוּ שָׁמָּה

Lo neida mah na'avod et Yah ad bo'einu shamah.

We don't know how we will serve God until we get there.
—Exodus 10:26 [11]

Prayer

Blessing for reading the Megillah:

בָּרוּךְ אַתָּה יְהֹוָה אֱלֹהֵינוּ מֶלֶךְ הָעוֹלָם אֲשֶׁר קִדְּשָׁנוּ בְּמִצְוֹתָיו וְצִוָּנוּ עַל מִקְרָא מְגִלָּה

Baruch atah Adonai, Eloheinu melech ha'olam,
asher kidshanu bamitzvotav, v'tzivanu al mikrah megillah.

Blessed are You, Adonai our God, Sovereign of the Universe, Who sanctifies us
with mitzvot and has commanded us to read the megillah.

Holiday Songs

מִשֶּׁנִּכְנַס אֲדָר מַרְבִּין בְּשִׂמְחָה

Mi she nichnas b'Adar, marbim b'simcha.

When the month of Adar begins, one increases rejoicing.
—Talmud / Ta'anit 29a

עַל הַנִּסִּים וְעַל הַפֻּרְקָן וְעַל הַגְּבוּרוֹת וְעַל הַתְּשׁוּעוֹת
וְעַל הַמִּלְחָמוֹת שֶׁעָשִׂיתָ לַאֲבוֹתֵינוּ בַּיָּמִים הָהֵם בַּזְּמַן הַזֶּה

Al hanisim, v'al hapurkan, v'al hagevurot, ve'al hateshuot, v'al hamilchamot
she'asitah la'avoteinu, ba'yamim hahem, ba'z'man hazeh.

For the miracles, for the redemption, for the mighty acts, for the consolations,
and for the battles that You performed for our foreparents, in those days, at
this time.

לַיְּהוּדִים הָיְתָה אוֹרָה וְשִׂמְחָה וְשָׂשׂוֹן וִיקָר כֵּן תִּהְיֶה לָנוּ תִּהְיֶה לָנוּ תִּהְיֶה לָנוּ

Layehudim hayetah orah v'simkhah v'sason v'ikar
Kein tihyeh lanu, tihyeh lanu, tihyeh lanu.

The Jews of old had light, happiness, joy, and love. May it be so for us.
—Esther 8:16

---

11. *The Power of Not-Knowing: Lo-Nayda,* https://www.rabbishefagold.com/power-of-not-knowing/

PASSOVER

Chant

קוּמִי לָךְ רַעְיָתִי יָפָתִי וּלְכִי לָךְ

Kumi lach rayati yafati ul'chi lach.

Arise my friend, oh beautiful one. Go to yourself.

—Song of Songs 2:10 [12]

Songs, Prayers, and Texts from the Haggadah

The Four Questions

מַה נִּשְׁתַּנָּה הַלַּיְלָה הַזֶּה מִכָּל הַלֵּילוֹת

Mah nishtanah halaylah hazeh mikol haleilot?

What makes this night different from all other nights?

On all other nights we eat chametz and matzah. Tonight, only matzah.

On all other nights we eat other vegetables. Tonight, only the bitter herb.

On all other nights, we don't dip our food even one time. Tonight, we dip it twice.

On all other nights, we eat either sitting or reclining. Tonight, we all recline.

Halachma Anyah

הָא לַחְמָא עַנְיָא דִּי אֲכָלוּ אַבְהָתָנָא בְּאַרְעָא דְמִצְרָיִם

Ha lachmah anyah di achalu avhatanah b'ar'ah d'Mitzrayim.

This is the bread of destitution that our ancestors ate in the land of Egypt.

Anyone who is famished, come and eat. Anyone who is in need, come partake of the Pesach sacrifice. Now we are here, next year we will be in the land of Israel. This year we are slaves, next year we will be free people.

Dayeinu

אִלּוּ הוֹצִיאָנוּ מִמִּצְרַיִם, דַּיֵּנוּ

Ilu hotziyanu mimitzra'im, dayeinu.

If God had taken us out of Egypt, it would have been enough for us.

אִלּוּ נָתַן לָנוּ אֶת־הַשַּׁבָּת, דַּיֵּנוּ

Ilu natan lanu et haShabbat, dayeinu.

If God had given us the Shabbat, it would have been enough for us.

אִלּוּ נַתַן לָנוּ אֶת־הַתּוֹרָה, דַּיֵּנוּ

Ilu natan lanu et haTorah, dayeinu.

If God had given us the Torah, it would have been enough for us.

---

12. *Arise My Friend: Kumi Lach,* https://www.rabbishefagold.com/arise-my-friend-kumi-lach/

L'shanah Haba'ah

לְשָׁנָה הַבָּאָה בִּירוּשָׁלָיִם

L'shanah haba'ah b'Yerushalayim!
Next year, let us be in Jerusalem!

COUNTING OF THE OMER

Chant

עָזִּי וְזִמְרָת יָהּ וַיְהִי לִי לִישׁוּעָה

Ozi v'zimrat Ya. Vay'hi li lishu'ah.
My strength balanced with the song of God will be my salvation.
—Psalm 118:14 [13]

Prayer

The Omer is counted every evening from the second night of Passover until the holiday of Shavuot. The blessing is as follows:

הִנְנִי מוּכָן וּמְזֻמָּן לְקַיֵּם מִצְוַת עֲשֵׂה שֶׁל סְפִירַת הָעֹמֶר. כְּמוֹ שֶׁכָּתוּב בַּתּוֹרָה

Hineni muchan um'zuman l'kayem mitzvat aseh shel s'firat ha'omer k'mo shekatuv baTorah:

Behold, I am ready and prepared to fulfill the mitzvah of counting the Omer, as it says in the Torah: You shall count from the eve of the second day of Pesach, when an Omer of grain is to be brought as an offering, seven complete weeks. The day after the seventh week of your counting will make 50 days.

בָּרוּךְ אַתָּה יְהֹוָה אֱלֹהֵינוּ מֶלֶךְ הָעוֹלָם אֲשֶׁר קִדְּשָׁנוּ בְּמִצְוֹתָיו וְצִוָּנוּ עַל סְפִירַת הָעֹמֶר

Baruch atah Adonai Eloheinu melech ha'olam
asher kid'shanu b'mitzvotav v'tzivanu al sefirat ha'omer.

Blessed are You, Adonai our God, Sovereign of the Universe,
Who sanctifies us with mitzvot and has commanded us to count the Omer.

After the blessing, one recites the day of the count:

הַיּוֹם יוֹם ___ לָעֹמֶר

Hayom, yom _____ la'omer
Today is the _____th day of the Omer,
marking ___ week(s) and ___ day(s) of the counting of the Omer.

---

13. *Balancing Will and Surrender: Ozi V'Zimrat Yah,* https://www.rabbishefagold.com/ozi-vzimrat-yah/

Chant

וְאֵרַשְׂתִּיךְ לִי לְעוֹלָם וְאֵרַשְׂתִּיךְ לִי בְּצֶדֶק וּבְמִשְׁפָּט וּבְחֶסֶד וּבְרַחֲמִים
וְאֵרַשְׂתִּיךְ לִי בֶּאֱמוּנָה וְיָדַעַתְּ אֶת־יְהוָה

V'eirastich li l'olam.
V'eirastich li b'tzedek uv'mishpat uv'chesed uv'rachamim.
V'eirastich li be'emunah v'yada'at et Adonai.

I will betroth you to Me forever. I will betroth you to Me with justice,
and with impeccability, and with love, and with compassion.
I will betroth you to Me in faith, and then you will know God.
—Hosea 2:21-22 [14]

Biblical Texts and Midrash

But Ruth replied, "Do not urge me to leave you, to turn back and not follow you.
For wherever you go, I will go. Wherever you lodge, I will lodge.
Your people shall be my people and your God my God."
—Ruth 1:16

The 10 Commandments

I, Adonai, am your God who brought you out of the land of Egypt, the house
of bondage.
You shall have no other gods besides Me.
You shall not swear falsely by the name of Adonai your God.
Remember the Sabbath day and keep it holy.
Honor your father and your mother.
You shall not murder.
You shall not commit adultery.
You shall not steal.
You shall not bear false witness against your neighbor.
You shall not covet anything that is your neighbor's.
—Exodus 20:1-14

When the Torah was given to the Children of Israel, they not only heard
God's Voice but actually saw the sound waves as they emerged from God's
mouth. They visualized them as a fiery substance. Each commandment that
left God's mouth traveled around the entire camp and then came back to
every Jew individually.
—Midrash / Shemot Rabbah 5:9

14. *Betrothal: V'Erestich-Li L'Olam,* https://www.rabbishefagold.com/betrothal/

When the Holy One gave the Torah, no bird chirped, no fowl fluttered, no ox lowed. The sea did not roar, the creatures did not speak. The universe was silent and mute. And the voice came forth: "I am Adonai, your God."
—Midrash / Exodus Rabbah 29:7

TISHA B'AV

Chant

וְהָפַכְתִּי אֶבְלָם לְשָׂשׂוֹן

V'hafachti evlam l'sason.
I will turn their mourning to joy.
—Jeremiah 31:13 [15]

Biblical Texts, Rabbinic Commentary, and Midrash

Between Kamtza and between Bar Kamtza, the Temple was destroyed.
—Midrash / Lamentations Rabbah 4:3 [16]

For My people have done a twofold wrong: They have forsaken Me, the Fount of Living Waters, and hewed them out cisterns, broken cisterns which cannot even hold water.
—Jeremiah 2:13 [17]

Once, Rabban Yohanan ben Zakkai was leaving Jerusalem and Rabbi Yehoshua, who was walking with him, took note of the ruined Temple. Rabbi Yehoshua said: "Woe is us on account of that which is ruined, that place in which we might atone for the sins of Israel!" Rabban Yohanan ben Zakkai replied: "My son, do not be troubled. We have another means of atonement." And what is that? *Gemilut hasadim,* deeds of loving kindness, as it is said, "For I desire kindness, not sacrifice."
—Hosea 6:6 and Avot d'Rabbi Natan, chapter 4

Holiday Song

עַל נַהֲרוֹת בָּבֶל שָׁם יָשַׁבְנוּ גַּם בָּכִינוּ בְּזָכְרֵנוּ אֶת־צִיּוֹן

Al naharot bavel sham yashavnu, gam bachinu b'zachreinu et Tziyon
By the rivers of Babylon, there we sat and wept, as we remembered Zion.
—Psalm 137:1

---

15. *Mourning into Joy: V'Hafachti,* https://www.rabbishefagold.com/mourning-into-joy/

16. It is taught that the Temple was destroyed not because of external enemies, but rather because of baseless hatred amongst Jews.

17. In the prophetic readings of "rebuke" that precede Tisha B'Av, Jeremiah warns the people that they must change their ways.

Chant

הֲשִׁיבֵנוּ יָה אֵלֶיךָ וְנָשׁוּבָה חַדֵּשׁ יָמֵינוּ כְּקֶדֶם

Hashiveinu Yah eileychah v'nashuvah. Hadeish yameinu k'kedem.

Now let us turn, return and be turned to the One!
—Lamentations 5:21 [18]

Songs and Prayers

Return again, return again. Return to the land of your soul.
Return again, return again. Return to the land of your soul.
Return to what you are. Return to who you are.
Return to where you are born and reborn again.
—Shlomo Carlebach

אַחַת שָׁאַלְתִּי מֵאֵת־יְהֹוָה אוֹתָהּ אֲבַקֵּשׁ
שִׁבְתִּי בְּבֵית־יְהֹוָה כָּל־יְמֵי חַיַּי
לַחֲזוֹת בְּנֹעַם־יְהֹוָה וּלְבַקֵּר בְּהֵיכָלוֹ:

Achat sha'alti mei'eit Adonai, otah avakeish
Shiviti b'veit Adonai kol y'mei chayay,
lachazot b'no'am Adonai ul'vakeir b'heichalo.

One thing I ask of Adonai, only that do I seek:
to live in the house of Adonai all the days of my life,
to gaze upon the beauty of Adonai, to frequent God's temple.
—Psalm 27:4 [19]

Biblical Text: Elul

אֱלוּל
אֲנִי לְדוֹדִי וְדוֹדִי לִי

Ani l'dodi v'dodi li.
I am my beloved's and my beloved is mine.
—Song of Songs 6:3

18. *Turn, Return, and Be Turned: Hashiveynu,* https://www.rabbishefagold.com/turn-return-and-be-turned/
19. This Psalm is offered throughout the month of Elul.

Glossary

Kabbalah (Hebrew) Meaning "that which is received," Kabbalah refers to the vast body of Jewish mystical, esoteric teachings that have evolved throughout centuries. The central text of Kabbalah is the *Zohar,* which was published in the 13th century.

Mantra (Sanskrit) Originating in Buddhism and Hinduism, a mantra is a sacred sound, word, phrase, or prayer that is repeated during meditation to heighten consciousness.

Midrash (Hebrew) From the Hebrew word *darash* which means to seek or to inquire, midrash is rabbinic interpretations that explain the relevance and meaning of particular Biblical passages.

Mishnah (Hebrew) Recorded in Aramaic (ancient spoken Hebrew) in the third century, the Mishnah is the first work of rabbinic literature, referred to as the Oral Torah, and forms the basis of *halacha* (religious law).

Mitzvah (Hebrew) Often translated "good deed," *mitzvah* literally means "commandment" (plural: *mitzvot*). There are 613 mitzvot found in Torah.

Pirke Avot (Hebrew) Translated as "The Chapters of the Fathers," Pirke Avot is comprised of terse ethical teachings from ancient rabbinic sages which are recorded in the Mishnah.

Pranayama (Sanskrit) These breathing techniques and exercises are used during the practice of yoga.

Sanskrit This is the ancient, classical language of India in which Hindu scriptures were written.

Talmud (Hebrew) The Talmud is the authoritative body of Jewish tradition comprising the Mishnah (see above) and the Gemara, which expands upon and clarifies the teachings of the Mishnah. Compiled in about 500 CE, the Talmud is comprised of 63 tractates. The Hebrew word *talmud* means "study."

Tanakh (Hebrew) This acronym refers to the three components of the Hebrew Bible: **T**orah, The Five Books of Moses; **N**evi'im, The Prophets; and **K**etuvim, The Writings.

Torah (Hebrew) Comprised of the Five Books of Moses: *Bereshit*, Genesis; *Shemot*, Exodus; *Vayikra*, Leviticus; *Bamidbar*, Numbers; and *Devarim*, Deuteronomy, the Torah is written on a scroll, housed in a synagogue's ark, and taken out to be read on Shabbat, weekdays, and holidays.

Yin Yang (Chinese) According to Taoist Chinese philosophy, these are two complementary yet opposing universal forces. Yin represents cool, dark, and slow characteristics whereas Yang embodies hot, bright, and fast attributes.

Yoga (Sanskrit) Originating in ancient India, yoga is the practice of physical postures, breathing exercises, and meditation to promote holistic health in body, mind, and spirit. Yoga encompasses a vast, complex body of knowledge based on physical, metaphysical, and philosophical teachings.

Jewish Yoga Community

Those seeking to create a bridge between Judaism and yoga represent a growing, international community. Join our journey. In-person retreats and training, along with virtual modes of gathering, are enabling new pathways for synergy and mutual support. Adapt this book to suit individual needs and curiosity about Judaism and yoga. Let us know your thoughts, ideas, insights, and questions.

- Email us at: levshalemyoga@gmail.com
- Visit our website at: www.LevShalemYoga.com

Jewish Yoga and Meditation Networks

- Jewish Yoga Network, www.jewishyoganetwork.org
- Embodied Jewish Learning, www.embodiedjewishlearning.org
- Institute for Jewish Spirituality, www.jewishspirituality.org
- The Awakened Heart Project, www.awakenedheartproject.org
- TorahYoga, www.torahyoga.com
- Rabbi Shefa Gold, www.rabbishefagold.com

Some Recommended Resources in Jewish Yoga and Meditation Books

Bloomfield, D.,*Torah Yoga: Experiencing Jewish Wisdom Through Classical Postures.* San Francisco, CA: Jossey-Bass, A Wiley Imprint, 2004.

Brotman, E., *Mussar Yoga: Blending an Ancient Jewish Spiritual Practice with Yoga to Transform Body and Soul.* Woodstock, VT: Jewish Lights Publishing, 2014.

Comins, M., *A Wild Faith: Jewish Ways into Wilderness, Wilderness Ways into Judaism.* Woodstock, VT: Jewish Lights Publishing, 2007.

Copeland, M., *I am the Tree of Life: My Jewish Yoga Book.* Millburn, NJ: Apples & Honey Press, 2020.

Dembe, S., *Wrestling with Yoga: Journey of a Jewish Soul.* USA., Shelly Dembe, 2013.

Frankiel, T., Greenfeld, J., *Minding the Temple of the Soul: Balancing Body, Mind, and Spirit Through Traditional Jewish Prayer, Movement, and Meditation.* Woodstock, VT: Jewish Lights Publishing, 1997.

Freed, M., *The Festive Sutras: A Yogi's Guide to Shabbat & Jewish Festivals.* Los Angeles, CA: Freedthinker Books, 2017.

Freed, M., *The Kabbalah Sutras: A Yogi's Guide to Counting the Omer.* Los Angeles, CA: Freedthinker Books, 2019.

Freed, M., *The Kosher Sutras: A Yogi's Guide to the Torah.* Los Angeles, CA: Freedthinker Books, 2013.

Gold, S., *Om Shalom: Yoga and Judaism. Explorations of a Jewish Yogi.* USA, Lulu Press, 2007.

Grunberger, L., *Yiddish Yoga: Ruthie's Adventures in Love, Loss, and the Lotus Position.* New York, NY: Newmarket Press, 2009.

Kamenetz, R., *The Jew in the Lotus.* New York, NY: Harper Collins, 1994.

Kaplan, A., *Jewish Meditation.* New York, NY: Schocken Books, 1985.

Levine, L., and Krucoff, C., *Yoga Shalom.* Millburn, NJ: Behrman House Books 2011

Lew, A., *Be Still and Get Going: A Jewish Meditation Practice for Real Life.* New York, NY: Little, Brown and Company, 2005.

Michaelson, J., *God in Your Body: Kabbalah, Mindfulness, and Embodied Spiritual Practice.* Woodstock, VT: Jewish Lights Publishing, 2007.

Roth, J., *Jewish Meditation Practices for Everyday Life: Awakening Your Heart, Connecting with God.* Woodstock, VT: Jewish Lights Publishing, 2009.

About the Authors and Illustrator

Rabbi Tara Feldman earned a BA in Russian Language and Literature from Vassar College, an MA in Elementary Education from Lesley College, and was ordained by Hebrew Union College in 2001. She served for more than a decade as co-senior rabbi of Temple Beth-El of Great Neck, New York; associate rabbi at Temple Israel in Memphis, Tennessee; rabbi educator at Congregation Beth Elohim in Brooklyn, New York; and was a fellow at Hebrew University's Melton Senior Educators program in Jerusalem. A Jew by choice, Rabbi Feldman's Jewish journey began with Rabbi Lawrence Kushner at Congregation Beth El in Sudbury, Massachusetts. A lifelong exercise enthusiast, her interests include yoga, meditation, and storytelling. Rabbi Feldman lives in Jerusalem, Israel, with her husband, Rabbi Meir Feldman, son and daughter.

Sharon Epstein earned a BA in Theater Arts from Bard College and an MS in Dance Movement Therapy from Hunter College. She has worked as a licenced creative arts therapist in the field of adult psychiatry, gerontology, oncology, and neurology. She started practicing yoga while in high school; yoga was then a complement to her movement studies. She completed her 200-hour training at the Yoga Polarity Center of Long Island and her 500-hour teacher training at Laughing Lotus in New York City. Sharon holds the credentials E-RYT-500 and YACEP from Yoga Alliance. As a yoga teacher and wellness coach, Sharon can be found leading individual, community and corporate programs in person and online. She loves empowering others to strengthen their Jewish roots and spiritual identity through yoga. Sharon lives in Great Neck, New York, with her husband, Ron. Together, they have raised two sons.

Adam J. Schiff attends the Art and Design High School in New York City. His work can be seen on Instagram at @schiffadamj and in the pages of Temple Beth-El of Great Neck's award-winning *Shema* magazine. Adam is also a musician and is working on the score to a production of *A Midsummer Night's Dream*. Adam plans to study art and music at college and is interested in continuing freelance work. He lives in New York City.

Made in United States
North Haven, CT
09 February 2022

15935674R10083